D1727485

With compliments:

 Diagnostics

Roche Diagnostics GmbH
Roche Laboratory Systems
D-68298 Mannheim
Germany

Iron Metabolism, Anemias

Diagnosis and Therapy

Novel concepts
in the anemias of renal
and rheumatoid disease

Fourth, enlarged edition

M. Wick
W. Pinggera
P. Lehmann

SpringerWienNewYork

Dr. Manfred Wick
Institute of Clinical Chemistry, Klinikum Grosshadern, University of Munich,
Germany

Prim. Univ.-Prof. Dr. Wulf Pinggera
Medical Department, General Hospital, Amstetten, Austria

Dr. Paul Lehmann
Roche Diagnostics Gmbh, Mannheim, Germany

Typesetting: Froschauer, A-3442 Langenrohr
Printing: Adolf Holzhausens Nachfolger, A-1070 Wien

Printed on acid-free and chlorine free bleached paper

With 54 Figures

ISBN 3-211-83357-9 Springer-Verlag Wien-New York
ISBN 3-211-82884-2 3rd ed. Spinger-Verlag Wien-New York

Foreword

Anemias are a worldwide problem. Severe anemia affects mainly the elderly. The WHO defines anemia as a hemoglobin concentration of less than 12 g/dl in women and less than 13 g/dl in men (World Health Organization. Nutritional Anemias. Technical Reports Series 1992; 503). According to these criteria 10 to 20 percent of women and 6 to 30 percent of men above the age of 65 years are anemic. In this book we place a new emphasis on the diagnosis and treatment of anemias of chronic disease (ACD) and renal anemias. Nevertheless, iron deficiency remains globally the most important cause of anemia.

There have been so many advances in the diagnosis and, in particular, the therapy of the anemias in recent years that it appeared necessary to extend the spectrum of therapies and diagnostic methods described. Apart from renal and inflammatory anemias, new insights regarding the role of transferrin receptor, the physiology of erythropoietin production and the genetic defect as well as the pathogenesis of hemochromatosis demanded a major update of the book.

The authors are grateful to Cheryl Byers, Annett Fahle and Kerstin Geiger of Roche Diagnostics, Heribert Bauer of Graphik-Art and Michael Katzenberger of the Springer-Verlag for their committed cooperation and their expert support in the publication of this book.

M. Wick
W. Pinggera
P. Lehmann

March 2000

Table of Contents

Introduction 1

Physiological Principles of Iron Metabolism and
  Erythropoiesis 3
  Absorption of Iron 3
  Iron Transport 5
    Transferrin and Iron-Binding Capacity 5
    Transferrin Saturation (TfS) 7
    Transferrin Receptor (TfR) 8
  Iron Storage 9
    Ferritin and Isoferritins 11
  Iron Distribution 13
  Iron Requirement... 13
  Iron Losses 16
  Erythropoiesis 16
    Physiological Cell Maturation 16
    Hemoglobin Synthesis 17
    Erythropoietin (EPO) 18
  Erythrocyte Degradation 21
    Phagocytosis of old Erythrocytes 21
    Hemoglobin Degradation 21

Disturbances of Iron Metabolism/
  Disturbances of Erythropoiesis and Hemolysis 23
  Disturbances of the Body's Iron Balance 23
  Iron Deficiency 25
  Iron Overload 27
    Primary Hemochromatosis 28
    Other Hereditary States of Iron Overload 30
  Disturbances of Iron Distribution 31
    Anemias of Chronic Diseases (ACD) in Inflammations 32
    Anemias of Malignancy 34

Disturbances of Iron Utilization 35
    Renal Anemias 36
    Pathophysiology of Erythropoietin Production 37
Non-iron-induced Disturbances of Erythropoiesis 39
    Disturbances of Stem Cell Proliferation 39
    Vitamin B_{12} and Folic Acid Deficiency 40
    Hemoglobinopathies 42
    Disturbances of Porphyrin Synthesis 45
Pathologically Increased Hemolysis 47
    Haptoglobin 47
    Features of Severe Hemolysis 48
    Causes of Hemolysis 49

**Diagnosis of Disturbances of Iron Metabolism/Disturbances
of Erythropoiesis** **51**
The Body's Iron Balance 51
    Iron Absorption Test 52
    Clinical Significance of the Determination of Ferritin 55
    Representative Ferritin Levels – Size of Iron Stores 56
    Transferrin, Transferrin Saturation 58
    Transferrin Receptor 60
Iron Deficiency and Decreased Ferritin Concentrations 63
    Prelatent Iron Deficiency 64
    Latent Iron Deficiency 64
    Manifest Iron Deficiency: Iron Deficient Anemia 65
    Differential Diagnosis of Iron Deficiency 65
    Clinical Pictures of Iron Deficiency 66
Iron Overload – Elevated Ferritin Concentrations 69
    Representative Ferritin Increase 70
    Primary Hemochromatosis 70
    Secondary Hemochromatosis 73
Disturbances of Iron Distribution 74
    Non-Representative Raised Plasma Ferritin Concentrations 74
    Anemia of Chronic Disorders (ACD) 75
    Iron and Cellular Immunity 76
    Iron, Acute-Phase Proteins, and Hormones 77
    Anemias of Rheumatoid Arthritis (RA) 77
    Anemias in Malignant Neoplasia (Erythropoietin as Tumor Marker) . 84
Disturbances of Iron Utilization 84
    Erythropoietin 85
    Uremic Anemia 86

Table of Contents

Non-iron-induced Disturbances of Erythropoiesis 87
Macrocytic Anemia 89
Folic Acid Deficiency 90
Vitamin B_{12} Deficiency 92
Normocytic Anemia 95
Extracorpuscular Hemolytic Anemias 95
Corpuscular Anemias 97
Deficiencies in the Cofactors of Erythropoiesis 97

Therapy of Anemias **105**
Therapy of Iron Deficiency 105
Oral Administration of Iron 105
Parenteral Administration of Iron 106
Side-effects and Hazards of Iron Therapy 108
Therapy of Iron Distribution Disorders 111
Anemia of Chronic Disease (ACD) 111
Rheumatoid Arthritis (RA) 111
Therapy of Chronic Inflammatory Processes 118
Therapy of Iron Utilization Disorders 120
Erythropoietin Deficiency,
Anemia in Renal Failure 120
Deficiencies in the Cofactors of Erythropoiesis 125
Vitamin B_{12} Deficiency 125
Folic Acid Deficiency 125
Autologous Blood Donors 126
Other Indications 126

Methods **127**
The Blood Count 127
Basic Tests of Hematopoiesis 128
Automated Cell Counting 129
The Impedance Principle 130
Flow Cytometry 131
Immunofluorescence 132
Hemoglobin (Hb) 135
Hematocrit (Hct) 137
Erythrocytes 138
Red Cell Count (RBC) 138
RBC Indices: MCV, MCH, MCHC 139
Reticulocytes 141
Reticulocyte Count 142

Reticulocyte Maturity Index (RMI) 142
Tests for the Diagnosis of Disorders of Iron Metabolism 144
Determination of Iron 146
   Iron Saturation = Total Iron-Binding Capacity (TIBC)
   and the Latent Iron-Binding Capacity (LIBC) 150
Determination of Iron-Binding Proteins: Immunoassay Methods 151
Ferritin 154
Transferrin (Tf) 158
   Relationship between Transferrin and
   Total Iron-Binding Capacity (TIBC) 160
   Transferrin Saturation (TfS) 160
Transferrin Receptor (TfR) 161
Haptoglobin 165
Ceruloplasmin (Cp) 166
Determination of Vitamin B_{12} and Folic Acid 167
   Vitamin B_{12} 168
   Folic Acid 170
Erythropoietin (EPO) 171
Tests for the Diagnosis of Chronic Inflammation (ACD) 174
Erythrocyte Sedimentation Rate (ESR) 175
C-Reactive Protein (CRP) 175
   CRP in Comparison with Other Acute Phase Reactants 177
Rheumatoid Factors (RF) 178
Iron/Copper Relation and Ceoruloplasmin 179

References 180

Recommended Reading 195

Subject Index 196

Introduction

Disturbances of iron metabolism, particularly iron deficiency and iron redistribution are among the most commonly overlooked or misinterpreted diseases. This is due to the fact that the determination of transport iron in serum or plasma, which used to be the conventional diagnostic test, does not allow a representative estimate of the body's total iron reserves. In the past a proper estimate was only possible by the costly and invasive determination of storage iron in the bone marrow. However, sensitive, well-standardized immuno-chemical methods for the precise determination of the iron storage protein ferritin in plasma are now available. Since the secretion of this protein correctly reflects the iron stores in the majority of cases, these methods permit fast and reliable diagnoses, particularly of iron deficiency status. In view of the high incidence of iron deficiency and its usually simple treatment, this fact should be common knowledge in the medical world.

Even non-iron-related causes of anemia can now be identified rapidly by highly sensitive, well standardized methods. We hope that this book will contribute to a better understanding of the main pathophysiological relationships and diagnostic principles (Fig. 1) of iron metabolism and anemias. However, the diagnosis of bone marrow diseases in the strict sense of the word, particularly if granulopoesis or thrombopoesis are involved, should remain the responsibility of hematologically experienced experts.

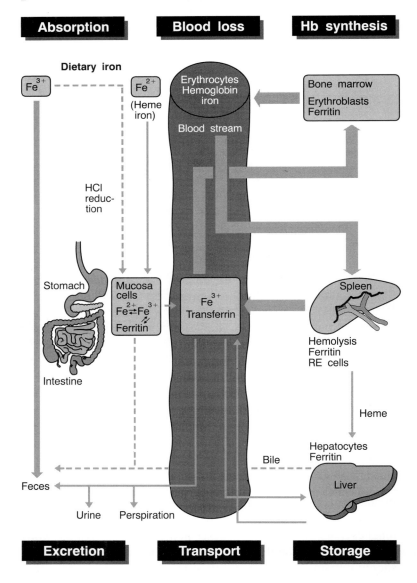

Fig. 1. Physiological principles of iron metabolism

Physiological Principles of Iron Metabolism and Erythropoiesis

Iron, as a constituent of hemoglobin and cytochromes, is one of the most important biocatalysts in the human body.

Absorption of Iron

The absorption of iron by the human body is limited by the physico-chemical and physiological properties of iron ions, and is possible only through protein binding of the Fe^{2+} ion (Fig. 2).

Iron is absorbed as Fe^{2+} in the duodenum and in the upper jejunum. Since iron in food occurs predominantly in the trivalent form it must (apart from the heme-bound Fe^{2+} component) first be reduced, e.g. by ascorbic acid (vitamin C). This explains why only about 10% of the iron in food, corresponding to about 1 mg per day, is generally absorbed. This daily iron intake represents only about 0.25 ‰ of the body's average total iron pool, which is approximately 4 g; this means that it takes some time to build up adequate reserves of iron. The actual iron uptake fluctuates considerably, depending on absorption-inhibiting and absorption-promoting influences in the upper part of the small intestine. The following factors inhibit absorption in clinically healthy individuals: reduced production of gastric acid, a low level of divalent iron as the result of an unbalanced diet (e.g., in vegetarians), a low level of reducing substances (e.g., ascorbic acid) in the food, or complex formation due to a high consumption of coffee or tea. Conversely, absorption is promoted by a combination of a meat-rich diet with a plentiful supply of heme-bound iron and an acidic, reducing environment due to a high consumption of fruit and vegetables.

The mechanism of iron absorption has become clearer recently. It is assumed to proceed in two stages. When they enter the cells of the mucosa, the Fe^{2+} ions are bound to transport sub-

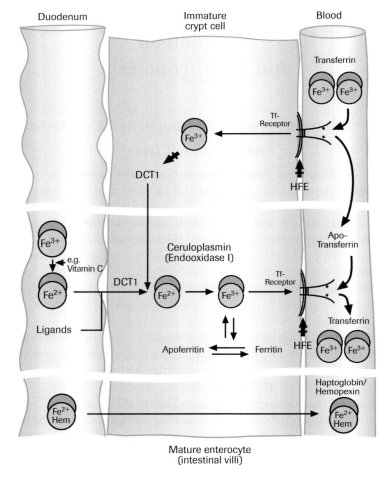

Fig. 2. Intestinal iron resorption (partially hypothetical)

stances like DCT1 (Divalent Cation Transporter) [47] . Before entering into the blood plasma they are oxidized to Fe^{3+} by endooxidase I (ceruloplasmin) and bound in this form to transferrin. Within certain limits, the absorption of iron can be adjusted to meet the current iron requirement. Iron deficiency, anemia, and hypoxia lead via increased transferrin and DCT1 synthesis to an increase in the absorption and transport capacity. Immature crypt cells serve as iron sensors by uptake of Fe^{3+} from plasma transferrin [137]. Low transferrin saturation increases DCT1 production. Conversely, the HFE protein limits iron uptake by transferrin receptor. Thereby, the cells of the mucosa protect the body against alimentary iron overload by storing surplus iron as ferritin; it is then excreted after a few days in the course of the physiological cell turnover. However, the physiological regulation mechanisms are unable to compensate for long-term extreme deviations of the iron supply; in particular, they are not sufficiently effective in severe diseases.

Iron Transport

Iron is normally transported via the specific binding of Fe^{3+} by transferrin in blood plasma [24]. The Fe^{3+}-transferrin complex in turn is bound by transferrin receptors to cells of the target organs which allows specific iron uptake according to the individual needs of the various cells. Pronounced non-specific binding to other transport proteins, such as albumin, occurs only in conditions of iron overload with high levels of transferrin saturation. Where there is an abundant supply of heme-bound iron, part of the Fe^{2+}-heme complex may escape oxidation in the cells of the mucosa and be transported to the liver after being bound by haptoglobin or hemopexin.

Transferrin and Iron-Binding Capacity

Transferrin is synthesized in the liver, and has a half-life of 8 to 12 days in the blood. It is a glycoprotein having a molecular weight of 79.6 kD, and β_1 electrophoretic mobility. Its synthesis in the liver may be increased as a corrective measure, depending on

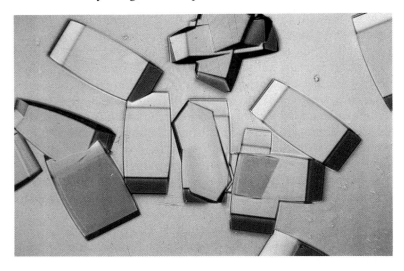

Fig. 3. Transferrin crystals [48]

iron requirements and iron reserves. At present little is known about the details of the regulatory mechanisms involved. Transferrin is detectable not only in blood plasma, but also in many interstitial fluids, and a locally synthesized variant with a low neuraminic acid content (β_2 or τ transferrin) is also found in the cerebrospinal fluid. The functional and immunological properties of the many isoforms are substantially the same, the only important difference being the isoelectric point [24]. These forms are therefore of no practical interest with regard either to analytical technique or to the assessment of the iron metabolism (except CDT: diagnosis of alcoholism and Beta-2-Transferrin: CSF diagnostics). Each transferrin molecule can bind a maximum of 2 Fe^{3+} ions, corresponding to about 1.41 µg of iron per mg of transferrin.

Since transferrin is the only specific iron transport protein, the total specific iron-binding capacity can be measured indirectly via the immunological determination of transferrin. In view of its practicability, its low susceptibility to interference,

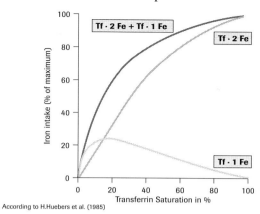

According to H.Huebers et al. (1985)

Fig. 4. Iron intake in the erythroid progenitor cell in dependency on transferrin saturation (TfS)

and its high specificity, this method should be used to determine the transferrin-bound iron transport. It has made the determination of the iron saturation = total iron-binding capacity (TIBC) and of the latent iron-binding capacity (LIBC) largely redundant. Under physiological conditions, transferrin is present in concentrations which exceed the iron-binding capacity normally necessary. About two thirds of the binding sites are therefore unoccupied. The fraction of transferrin binding sites that are not occupied by iron is known as the latent iron-binding capacity (LIBC). It is calculated from the difference between the total iron-binding capacity and the serum iron concentration.

Transferrin Saturation (TfS)

This procedure has been replaced by the determination of the percentage saturation of transferrin, which does not include non-specific binding of iron by other proteins, so that only the physiologically active iron binding is measured. Fluctuations of the transferrin concentration that are not due to regulatory mechanisms of the iron metabolism can also be eliminated from the assessment in this manner.

Approximately one third of the total iron-binding capacity is normally saturated with iron. Whereas the transferrin concentration remains constant in the range from 2.0 to 4.0 g/l, without any appreciable short-term fluctuations, the transferrin saturation changes quickly with the iron concentration depending on the time of day, the current iron requirement, and the intake of iron in food. The total quantity of transferrin-bound transport iron in the blood plasma of a healthy adult is only about 4 mg, i.e. only 1 ‰ of the body's total iron pool.

It is clear from the very low plasma iron concentration and its short-term fluctuations that neither the plasma iron concentration nor the transferrin saturation can provide a true picture of the body's total iron reserves. Assessment of the body's iron reserves is only possible by determination of the storage protein ferritin.

The plasma iron concentration and the transferrin saturation only become relevant in the second stage of diagnosis for differentiation of conditions with high plasma ferritin concentrations (see "Disturbances of Iron Distribution"). The determination of the transferrin saturation is preferable to the determination of iron alone, since this eliminates the effects of different blood sampling techniques, different states of hydration of the patient, and different transferrin concentrations.

Transferrin Receptor (TfR)

All tissues and cells which require iron regulate their iron uptake by expression of the transferrin receptor on the surface of the cell. Since most of the iron is required for hemoglobin synthesis in the precursor cells of erythropoiesis in the bone marrow, approximately 80% of the transferrin receptors of the body can be found on these cells. All cells are capable of regulating individual transferrin receptor expression according to the current iron requirement or the supply of iron at the cell level. A small but representative proportion of these transferrin receptors is also released into the blood as so-called soluble transferrin receptors and can be detected by immunochemical methods in a concentration of a few milligrams per liter. It is a dimeric protein with a molecular weight of approximately 190 000 daltons, each of the two sub-units is capable of binding a molecule of transferrin [134].

In iron metabolism the transferrin receptor has a major role in supplying the cell with iron. Fe ion transport in the blood occurs by the specific binding of Fe^{3+} ions to transferrin; a maximum of two Fe^{3+} ions can be transported per protein molecule. The affinity of the membrane-bound transferrin receptor to the transferrin-Fe complex in the weakly alkaline pH of the blood depends on the Fe load of the transferrin. A maximum is reached when the Tf load is 2 Fe ions.

The TfR-Tf-Fe complex is channeled through a pH gradient into the cell by the "endocytic residue". The change from the alkaline pH of the blood to the acidic pH of the endosome changes the binding situation: Iron ions dissociate spontaneously from the transferrin while the bond between Tf and TfR is strengthened. Only when the TfR-Tf complex returns to the cell membrane does the pH change there cause the complex to dissociate. The transferrin reenters the plasma and is again available for Fe transport.

Expression of the transferrin receptor is regulated by the intracellular concentration of the iron ions. If the iron requirement of the cell is large, but the iron concentration is small, TfR expression and, at the same time, the concentration of the soluble serum transferrin receptor increases. Conversely, where there is iron overload, both the TfR concentration and the concentration of soluble TfR are low.

As the concentration of the soluble transferrin receptor reflects the total number of cell-bound transferrin receptors and these, in turn, are mainly to be found on erythropoietic cells in the bone marrow, in a healthy person with an adequate iron supply the transferrin-receptor concentration is one of the best indicators of erythropoietic activity [8, 59, 134].

Iron Storage

Because of the very limited iron absorption capacity, the average iron requirement can only be met by extremely economical recycling of active iron. Iron is stored in the form of ferritin or its semi-crystalline condensation product hemosiderin in the liver, spleen, and bone marrow [37]. In principle, every cell has the ability to store an excess of iron through ferritin synthesis. The fundamental mechanisms are identical for all types of cells (Fig. 5).

The transferrin-Fe^{3+} complex is bound to the transferrin receptor of the cell membrane. Iron uptake can therefore be regulated by the transferrin receptor expression [20]. Iron directly induces the synthesis of apoferritin, the iron-free protein shell of ferritin, on the cytoplasmic ribosomes. In the majority of metabolic situations, a representative fraction of the ferritin synthesized is released into the blood plasma [37]. The ferritin concentration correctly reflects the amount of storage iron available *(exception:* disturbances of iron distribution). This has been verified experimentally by comparison with iron determinations in bone-marrow aspirates [40, 68]. In clinical diagnosis ferritin should be determined as the parameter of first choice for the assessment of iron reserves, e.g. in the identification of the cause of an anemia.

The relationship between iron reserves and serum ferritin is valid for all stages of iron deficiency, the normal state and all forms of iron overload in the absence of any significant subsequent organ damage. 1 ng/ml of serum ferritin corresponds to approximately 10 mg of stored iron. This can be used not only to estimate the amount of iron required to replenish stores during iron deficiency but also to estimate iron excess in the case of iron overload as well as for the monitoring of the course of these disorders.

In addition to the general mechanisms of cellular iron storage and uptake, the liver and the spleen also have specialized metabolic pathways. Hepatocytes, for example, can convert haptoglobin-bound or hemopexin-bound hemoglobin-Fe^{2+} or heme-Fe^{2+} from intravascular hemolysis or from increased heme absorption into ferritin-Fe^{3+} storage in iron. On the other hand, the regular lysis of senescent erythrocytes and the associated conversion of Fe^{2+}-hemoglobin into Fe^{3+}-ferritin storage iron takes place mainly in the reticuloendothelial cells of the spleen. The re-export of Fe from storage cells and binding to transferrin requires an intracellular oxidation by ceruloplasmin (= endooxidase I), which is deficient in acoeruloplasminaemia.

Ferritin and Isoferritins

Ferritin is a macromolecule having a molecular weight of at least 440 kD (depending on the iron content), and consists of a protein shell (apoferritin) of 24 subunits and an iron core containing an average of about 2500 Fe^{3+} ions (in liver and spleen ferritin) (Fig. 5). Ferritin tends to form stable oligomers (approx. 10 to 15%), and when present in excess in the cells of the storage organs it tends to condense, with formation of semi-crystalline, microscopically visible hemosiderin in the lysosomes, which can be used diagnostically.

At least 20 isoferritins can be distinguished using isoelectric focusing [3] (Fig. 6). The microheterogeneity is due to differences in the contents of acidic H subunits and slightly basic L subunits.

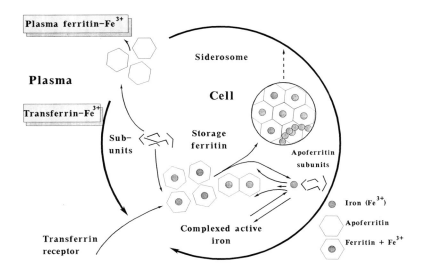

Fig. 5. Scheme of Cellular iron storage and ferritin synthesis
(DCT 1: Divatent Cation Transporter) [47]

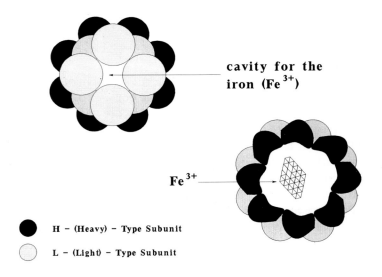

Fig. 6. Structure of the ferritin molecule

The basic isoferritins are responsible for long-term iron storage, and are found mainly in the liver, spleen, and bone marrow. The storage ferritins of this group can be measured by the commercially available immunoassay methods, which are standardized against liver and/or spleen ferritin preparations. Their determination provides a reliable picture of the iron reserves [22]. A new standardization based on a recombinant L-ferritin standard is in progress.

Acidic isoferritins are found mainly in myocardium, placenta, and tumor tissue, and in smaller quantities also in the depot organs. They have lower iron contents, and presumably function as intermediaries for the transfer of iron in synthetic processes [62]. Unlike the basic isoferritins, they exhibit practically no response to the commercially available immunoassay methods. The use of suitable highly specific antisera would be necessary for their selective determination (Fig. 7).

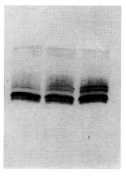

1. Heart ferritin
2. Liver ferritin
3. Spleen ferritin

3 2 1

Fig. 7. Isoelectric focusing of acidic (top) and basic isoferritins (bottom)

Iron Distribution

It can be seen from Fig. 9 that most (about 2500 mg) of the total iron pool is contained in the erythrocytes as hemoglobin-bound active iron. A further 400 mg is required as active iron in myoglobin and various enzymes. If the supply of iron is adequate (men and postmenopausal women), considerable quantities are also stored as basic ferritin (approx. 800 to 1200 mg) in the depot organs liver, spleen, and bone marrow [37]. Only a small fraction (approx. 4 mg) of the body's total iron pool is in the form of transferrin-bound transport iron in the blood plasma. It is thus once again clear that the measurement of iron in plasma does not provide a true picture of the available storage iron.

Iron Requirement

The iron distribution described is valid only for healthy adult men and for postmenopausal women, who have an iron replacement requirement of not more than 1 mg per day. The iron requirement is up to 5 mg per day for adolescents, menstruating women, pregnant women, and blood donors, as well as in cases of extreme physical stress due to anabolic processes or iron losses. This increased requirement cannot always be met by in-

Ferritin

Iron storage protein
Molecular weight ≥ 440 kD

Isoferritins

Basic isoferritins	Acidic isoferritins
Rich in iron	Poor in iron
Liver	Placenta
Spleen	Heart
Bone marrow	Tumors

Plasma ferritin is basic and correlates with the body's total iron stores (exception: disturbances of iron distribution)

Fig. 8. Clinically important characteristics of ferritin

creased absorption, even with an adequate supply of iron in the food. The result is a progressive depletion of the iron stores, which can lead to manifest iron deficiency if the supply of iron remains inadequate over a long period.

Where iron requirement is increased for the reasons given above, transferrin receptor expression is up-regulated. At the same time the concentration of the soluble transferrin receptor in the plasma rises accordingly. In most cases, increased erythropoiesis is the main reason for the increased iron requirement. However, it remains to be emphasized that the internal iron demand for Hb synthesis (25 mg) by far exceeds the average daily absorption and excretion of about 1 mg.

Iron Losses

A total of about 1 mg of iron per day is excreted via the intestine, urine and perspiration. Menstruating women lose 30 to 60 ml of

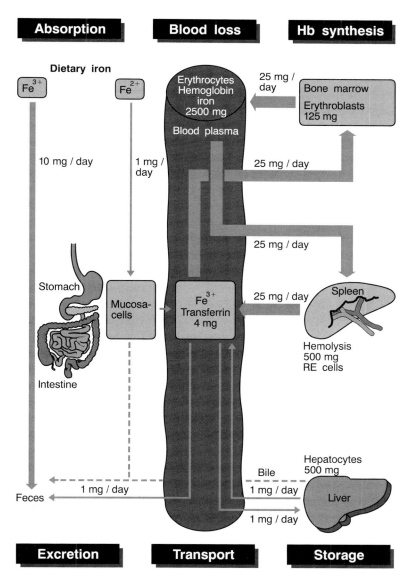

Fig. 9. Balance of iron metabolism

Steady-state

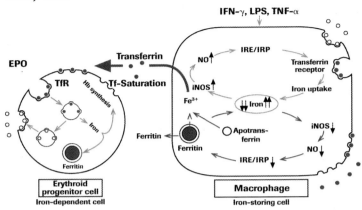

Fig. 10. Model of the autoregulatory loop between iron metabolism and the NO/NOS pathway in activated monocytes/macrophages and supply of an iron dependent cell. [140,142]

Abbreviations: IFN-γ, interferon γ; iNOS = inducible nitric oxide synthase; IRE, iron-responsive element; IRE/IRP high-affinity binding of iron-regulatory protein (IRP) to IREs; LPS, lipopolysaccharide; TNF-α, tumor necrosis factor α; ↑ and ↓ indicate increase or decrease of cellular responses, respectively.

Explanation of signs:
  ⌣ transferrin receptor,   ● iron-carrying transferrin,
  ○ apotransferrin,   ⊙ ferritin.

Iron stored as ferritin within an iron-storing cell is released and bound to apotransferrin, followed by its transport to the iron-dependent cell. The cytoplasmic membrane contains transferrin receptors to which the iron-carrying transferrin binds. The endosome migrates into the cytoplasm where it releases iron. The free iron is either used as functional iron or is stored as ferritin. The endosome returns to the cytoplasmic membrane and apotransferrin is released into the extracellular space.

blood, containing about 15 to 30 mg of iron, every month. With an adequate supply of iron in the diet, these losses can be replaced through increased absorption.

Hypermenorrhea, particularly in combination with an unbalanced diet, is a cause of iron deficiency. Another cause is frequent blood donations.

Erythropoiesis

Physiological Cell Maturation

An adult has on average 5 liters of blood and an erythrocyte count of 5 x 10^6/µl, giving a total erythrocyte count of 2.5 x 10^{13}. Since the mean life span of an erythrocyte is normally 120 days, about 2 x 10^{11} new erythrocytes need to be formed daily to maintain this erythrocyte pool. For this to happen, about 20-30% of the medullary stem cells must be differentiated to cells of erythropoiesis. Different stages in maturation can be identified on the basis of cell morphology and biochemical capacity. The immature nucleated cells, such as proerythroblasts and erythroblasts (macroblasts), with their high DNA, RNA and protein synthesizing capacity, ensure that there is adequate proliferation of erythrocyte precursors under stimulation by erythropoetin.

However, this requires the availability of sufficient cobalamin (vitamin B_{12}) and folic acid, which act as carriers of C_1 units in the synthesis of nucleic acids. Vitamin B_{12} (daily requirement about 2 µg) is derived mainly from foods of animal origin. Absorption in the terminal ileum calls for production of sufficient intrinsic factor by the parietal cells in the fundus/body region of the stomach. By contrast, folic acid (daily requirement > 200 µg) is derived mainly from foods of plant origin and, probably for the most part, via synthesis by intestinal bacteria, and absorbed in the jejunum. Considerable amounts of both vitamins are stored in the liver.

Hemoglobin synthesis then occurs at the normoblast stage of maturation, which is shown morphologically in the conversion of so-called basophilic into oxyphilic normoblasts (with red cytoplasm). Once the normoblast is filled with hemoglobin, the cell nucleus and mitochondria can be expelled, and the cell which leaves the bone marrow is known as a reticulocyte. It thereby loses most of its biochemical synthesis capabilities and its ability to divide, and subsequently circulates in the peripheral blood as a highly specialized, mature erythrocyte serving almost exclusively for the transportation of oxygen. All forms of anemia that are not primarily hemolytic thus have their roots in disturbances of cell proliferation or hemoglobin synthesis or in deficiencies at bone-marrow level.

Hemoglobin Synthesis

Hemoglobin consists of over 90% protein; in the fetus this is made up of 2α- and 2γ-polypeptide chains (known as HbF), whereas in adults it is predominantly 2α- and 2β-chains (HbA$_0$), with a small portion of 2α- and 2δ-chains (HbA$_2$).

Each of these chains carries a heme as prosthetic group, which in turn is capable of binding an oxygen molecule. The total molecular weight of this tetramer is about 68,000 D.

The formation of the normal quaternary structure is dependent on the regular synthesis not only of the protein chains but also of the porphyrin component, and in particular on the adequate adhesion of the heme and protein components by means of iron which also guarantees oxygen binding [119]. An overview of hemoglobin synthesis is given in Fig. 11.

Erythropoietin (EPO)

Erythropoietin (EPO) is a glycoprotein with a molecular weight of 34,000 daltons (Fig. 12). As hematopoietic growth factor, the hormone regulates the rate of red cell-production, keeping the circulating red cell mass constant. EPO is produced in response to a hypoxia signal as a result of a decrease in the oxygen tension in the blood.

This hormone, which is produced primarily in the kidney, stimulates the proliferation of the bone marrow erythroid pro-

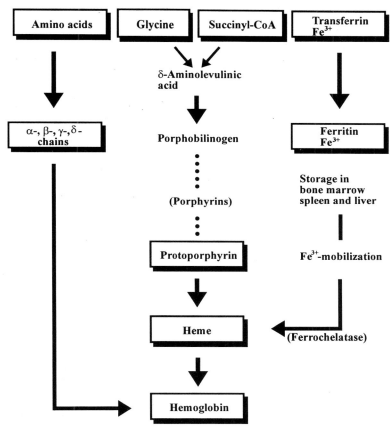

Fig. 11. Hemoglobin synthesis

genitor cells, accelerates their differentiation into mature erythrocytes, promotes hemoglobin synthesis and TfR expression
[140] and stimulates the release of reticulocytes from the bone
marrow (Fig. 13).

Up to now the determination of erythropoietin has been of
limited diagnostic value. It can be used, for example, to differentiate between primary causes of erythrocytosis such as
polycythemia vera and secondary causes such as increased pro-

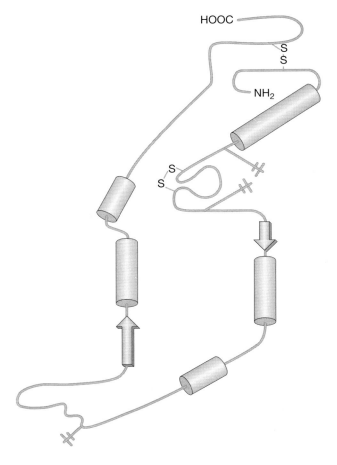

Fig. 12. Molecular biology of erythropoietin [from: Wieczorek K, Hirth P, Schöpe KB, Scigalla P, Krüger D (1989). In: Gurland S (ed), Innovative Aspekte der klinischen Medizin. Springer, Berlin Heidelberg New York Tokyo, pp 55-70]

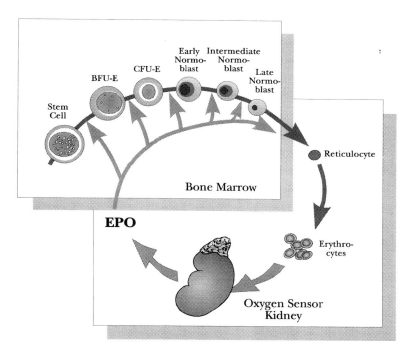

Fig. 13. Stimulation and regulation of erythrocyte formation by erythropoietin

duction of erythropoietin, e.g. in lung diseases with hypoxia or certain tumors. In renal anemia, decreased erythropoietin production can usually be assumed to be the cause. In anemia of chronic disease an inadequate erythropoietin response, that is anemia with normal erythropoietin levels, may be one of the main causes. In anemia of uncertain origin determination of erythropoietin can help to detect cases which are caused by insufficient erythropoietin production (see "Pathophysiology of Erythropoietin Production").

Erythrocyte Degradation

Phagocytosis of old Erythrocytes

During the physiological aging process the circulating erythrocytes lose more and more of the terminal neuraminic acid residues of their membrane glycoproteins, which leads to increased binding of IgG. This changed membrane surface structure is now the signal to the macrophages of above all the spleen and the liver to start phagocytosis of the old erythrocytes. This occurs physiologically after about 120 days, so that 0.8% of the erythrocyte pool or 2×10^{11} erythrocytes are lysed each day, maintaining equilibrium with the daily new formation rate.

Hemoglobin Degradation

The globin component of the hemoglobin is hydrolyzed by proteases to amino acids which are either available for the synthesis of new proteins or are further degraded by deamination. The iron which is released must be reused extremely economically and, so as to avoid toxic effects, oxidized and incorporated into basic isoferritins for interim storage. In this process, the macrophages of the RES (reticuloendothelial system) in particular in the spleen serve as short-term stores from which ferritin-bound iron can be remobilized and transported via transferrin to the bone marrow for the synthesis of new hemoglobin. At a physiological hemolysis rate, about 6.5 g per day of hemoglobin is catabolized, and the corresponding quantity newly synthesized, giving an iron turnover of about 25 mg/24 h [113, 119]. Given a daily iron absorption of 1 mg, this again shows clearly that the iron requirement can be met only after careful reutilization. The porphyrin ring of the heme is degraded to bilirubin via biliverdin. Since nonglucuronidized bilirubin is not water-soluble, it must first be transported in albumin-bound form to the liver where it is conjugated with glucuronic acid and thus converted into a form which can be eliminated with the bile (Fig. 14).

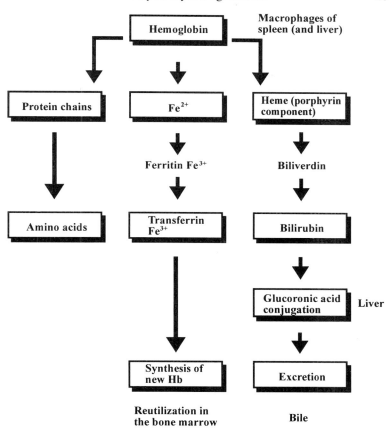

Fig. 14. Hemoglobin degradation

Disturbances of Iron Metabolism/ Disturbances of Erythropoiesis and Hemolysis

Disturbances of the Body's Iron Balance

An impaired iron balance of the body can frequently be described as a discordant regulation of synthesis of ferritin, the iron storage protein, on the one hand, and of the transferrin receptor, the indicator of iron demand and erythropoietic activity, on the other. This is particularly true if iron deficiency or iron overload are not complicated by additional diseases such as inflammations, tumors or renal failure (Table 1).

In true storage iron deficiency a lack of intracellular iron ions leads to downregulation of apoferritin synthesis and consequently also to a decreased release of ferritin into the peripheral blood. To compensate for this, expression of transferrin receptor is upregulated in order to meet the iron demand of the cell despite depleted iron reserves and low transferrin saturation. This leads to an increased concentration of soluble transferrin receptor in blood. This discordant regulation may be found already in latent iron deficiency, preceding the development of a hypochromic anemia. If these changes are not yet very marked, in doubtful cases the ratio of transferrin receptor and ferritin concentrations may show this state more clearly. The transport iron, determined by measuring the transferrin saturation, additionally contributes to the staging.

Opposite dysregulations are found in simple iron overload (for instance hereditary hemochromatosis) unless associated with

Table 1. Ferritin versus soluble transferrin receptor (sTfR)

Disease	Ferritin Iron stores	s TfR Iron needs
Iron deficiency	↓	↑
Iron overload	↑	n - ↓ (except hemolysis)
Iron redistribution (ACD)	↑	n
Iron utilization defects (incl. MPS, MDS)	n - ↑	n - ↑ (except renal and aplastic anemia)
Hemolysis	n - ↑	↑
Renal anemia (without EPO)	n - ↑	↓
Aplastic anemia	↑	↓

chronic inflammations, malignant disease, ineffective erythropoiesis or hemolysis. In cases of simple iron overload increase of ferritin and downregulation of transferrin receptor are delayed because induction of these regulatory mechanisms requires a significant accumulation of intracellular iron. Therefore, particularly in hereditary hemochromatosis increased transferrin saturation may be the most sensitive parameter for early detection, apart from PCR.

This discordant regulation of ferritin and transferrin receptor production is impaired, however, in cases of iron redistribution in chronic inflammations or tumors, in cases of increased erythropoietic activity due to hemolysis or erythropoietin therapy or in bone marrow diseases with increased but ineffective erythropoiesis (for instance myelodysplastic syndrome). This unusual reaction pattern can, however, be used to diagnose an increased iron demand despite sufficient or even increased iron reserves, particularly under erythropoietin therapy.

Iron Deficiency

Under physiological conditions, an increased iron requirement and/or increased loss of iron (in puberty, in menstruating or pregnant women, in blood donors or in competitive athletes) can lead to iron deficiency. With an unbalanced diet, the iron balance is often upset by a shortage of absorbable iron.

The first stage is a shortage of depot iron (prelatent iron deficiency), which is reflected in a reduced plasma ferritin concentration. When the iron stores are completely empty, a transport iron deficiency develops, though hemoglobin synthesis is still adequate at this stage (latent iron deficiency). With additional stress or loss of iron, however, this condition may progress into a manifest iron deficiency with hypochromic microcytic anemia. The latter is more often associated with a pathological chronic loss of blood, especially as a result of ulcers or tumors of the gastrointestinal and urogenital tracts, or with disturbances of iron absorption (e.g., after resections in the upper gastrointestinal tract) or chronic inflammatory diseases of the small intestine.

All forms of iron deficiency can be identified by the following pattern of laboratory findings: reduced ferritin concentration with a compensating increase in the transferrin concentration and low transferrin saturation (see "Diagnostic Strategies"). The reduced ferritin concentration is the only reliable indicator of iron-deficient conditions. It enables the latter to be distinguished from other causes of hypochromic anemia, such as chronic inflammations and tumors [55] (Table 2).

Iron deficiency, of whatever cause, also leads to increased transferrin receptor expression and accordingly to an increased concentration of the soluble transferrin receptor in the plasma. In these cases there is no longer any correlation between transferrin receptor and erythropoietic activity. Most forms of depot iron deficiency can be detected with an adequate degree of certainty by a decreased ferritin concentration.

However, in iron deficiency due to bleeding, inflammations or tumors this may be masked. On the other hand, in cases with

Table 2. Characteristic changes in parameters accompanying disturbances of iron metabolism ($\uparrow$ = increased, $\downarrow$ = decreased, n = normal)

	Ferritin	Transferrin	Iron	Transferrin saturation	Blood count and other findings
Iron deficiency	$\downarrow$	$\uparrow$	n - $\downarrow$	$\downarrow$	Hypochromic anemia
Disturbance of distribution of iron	$\uparrow$	n - $\downarrow$	n - $\downarrow$	n - $\downarrow$	Hypochromic anemia
Tumor inflammation	(Ferritin $\uparrow$ falsely indicates iron overload)				
Iron overload Hemolysis	$\uparrow$	n - $\downarrow$	n - $\uparrow$	n - $\uparrow$	Reticulocytes $\uparrow$ Signs of hemolysis
Ineffective erythropoiesis	$\uparrow$	n - $\downarrow$	n - $\uparrow$	n - $\uparrow$	Reticulocytes $\downarrow$ Blood count according to primary disease
Iatrogenetic iron overload, e.g. after multiple transfusions	$\uparrow$	$\downarrow$	$\uparrow$	$\uparrow$	Blood count depends on primary disease Secondary organic lesions
Hemochromatosis	$\uparrow$	$\downarrow$	$\uparrow$	$\uparrow$	Signs of secondary organic lesions

sufficient iron reserves and only so-called functional iron deficiency, i.e. disturbances of iron utilization, an increasing concentration of soluble transferrin receptors may give an early indication of the relative shortage of iron of erythropoiesis or deficient iron mobilization (see also "Disturbances in Iron Utilization in Dialysis Patients"). In these cases of complicated storage or functional iron deficiency, sTfR may show the increased iron demand.

Iron Overload

Genuine iron overload situations arise either through a biologically inappropriate increase in the absorption of iron despite adequate iron reserves, or iatrogenically as a result of frequent blood transfusions or inappropriate iron therapy [55].

The former condition occurs mainly as a result of the disturbance of negative feedback mechanisms, which in hemochromatosis is manifested as a failure of the protective mechanism in the mucosa cell due to a defective HFE protein.

Conditions characterized by ineffective erythropoiesis, such as MDS, thalassemia, porphyrias, and sideroachrestic as well as hemolytic anemias, presumably lead to increased absorption of iron as result of hypoxia, despite adequate or even increased iron reserves. The iron overload in these cases is aggravated by the necessary transfusions and by the body's inability to actively excrete iron. All the mechanisms mentioned ultimately lead to overloading of the iron stores, and hence redistribution to the parenchymal cells of many organs, such as the liver, heart, pancreas, and gonads. The storage capacity of the ferritin synthesis or of the lysosomes may thus be exceeded. The release of free iron ions and lysosomal enzymes has a toxic effect.

The toxic effects of iron overload are due to the presence of free iron ions which are able to form oxygen radicals. The main manifestations in these organs are toxic liver damage with liver cirrhosis and primary liver cell carcinoma, heart failure, diabetes or impotence. New investigations also show that phagocytosis and oxidative burst of granulocytes and monocytes may be impaired. Apart from this, epidemiological investigations have revealed iron overload to be a risk factor for atherosclerosis due to increased oxidation of lipoproteins.

This calls for an increased surveillance of iron overload in the latent phase already by regular ferritin determinations. This is true not only for primary hemochromatosis or secondary hemosiderosis and hematological disease but particularly also in patients with renal anemia or anemia of chronic disease under erythropoietin and iron substitution.

All genuine iron overload conditions are recognizable by elevated plasma ferritin concentrations together with elevated iron levels and increased transferrin saturation values, usually with a compensating decrease in transferrin synthesis. The increased transferrin saturation, as a sign of increased iron turnover and iron transport, distinguishes iron overload from conditions with redistribution of iron and non-representatively raised plasma ferritin concentrations.

Transferrin receptor expression can vary, depending on the reason for the iron overload, in particular whether erythropoiesis is increased or decreased. Correspondingly there is also an elevated transferrin receptor concentration in the plasma in all hemolytic conditions with raised erythropoietic activity.

Contrary to this, all bone marrow disorders with reduced erythropoiesis such as aplastic anemia and also renal failure (without erythropoietin therapy) are characterized by reduced transferrin receptor expression. Erythropoiesis is not directly affected in hemochromatosis. Transferrin receptor expression may be normal or decreased [134].

Primary Hemochromatosis

Primary hemochromatosis represents the most important form of hereditary iron overload. Up till now its significance has been underestimated but nevertheless a close association between primary hemochromatosis and certain HLA patterns has been known about for quite some time. Recently two mutations of the HLA-H gene or the HFE gene were discovered and have been found in the majority of white hemochromatosis patients in the homozygous or complementary heterozygous form. The cys-282-tyr mutation is by far the most common mutation and is present in homozygous form in almost 100% of Scandinavian hemochromatosis patients and as many as 69% of Italian hemochromatosis patients. The less common variant is the his-63-asp mutation. Both variations together represent probably the most common of all genetic defects. In the Caucasian population the frequency of the heterozygous defect is 1:15 and that of the homozygous form 1:200 to 1:300 [112].

The mutations obviously give rise to an abnormal HFE protein in the epithelial cells of the mucosa of the small intestine in the region which is relevant for iron absorption. It has been known for quite some time that an inadequately elevated iron resorption represents a major pathomechanism in the development of hemochromatosis. Mutated HFE proteins lead to an inadequately elevated iron absorption and therefore a failure of the protective mechanism in mucosal cells by a failure to inhibit the transferrin receptor. As a result, the negative feedback, which normally decreases DCT1 production and the binding of Fe^{3+} to Transferrin at already high Tf saturation, is compromised.

While usually only homozygous patients develop manifest hemochromatosis, even heterozygous patients have increased iron absorption and ferritin values.

Not all patients who have a homozygous gene defect actually develop manifest hemochromatosis. The frequency of hemochromatosis in the Caucasian population is in the order of 1:1000 to 1:2000. This is probably primarily due to the fact that the precondition for clinical manifestation of hemochromatosis is iron overloading of approximately 10-20 g corresponding to serum ferritin values of approximately 1000-2000 ng/ml. Assuming a positive iron balance of approximately 1 mg per day (f.i. 2 mg absorption, 1 mg excretion), the time required for the accumulation of an appropriate excess of iron reserves is approximately 30-60 years. This correlates well with the main age of manifestation in men (35-55 years of age). Although the homozygous gene defect is more commonly found in women than men as a result of an evolutionary natural selection process, these women are mostly protected from the development of hemochromatosis until at least the onset of menopause. This is due to the fact that the excess iron absorption is approximately compensated for by iron loss of the same order of magnitude (15-30 mg) in the course of menstrual bleeding. Therefore the process of iron accumulation and iron over-loading in women with homozygous hemochromatic genes only commences at the onset of menopause and (compared to the process occurring in men) is delayed by decades into old age. Accordingly only about 10% patients with symptomatic hemochromatosis are women. In an evolutionary context this means that hemochromatic genes probably represent a natural selection advantage because they protect women against severe iron deficiency until at least the onset of menopause. Only after achievement of a significantly longer life-expectancy does iron accumulation prove to be disadvantageous.

The genetic defect can now be identified in the course of routine diagnostic procedures. These days PCR detection of the appropriate mutations represents the second level in hematochromatosis diagnostics after ferritin and transferrin saturation screening. Assaying for ferritin remains the decisive determination for the monitoring of iron reserves.

Other Hereditary States of Iron Overload

New insights have been gained concerning the role of ceruloplasmin in iron metabolism. This copper transporting protein seems to be important for intracellular oxidation of Fe^{2+} to Fe^{3+} which is necessary for release of iron ions from the cells and the binding to transferrin. This is exemplified by the very rare hereditary aceruloplasminemia where the lack of iron oxidation prevents binding to transferrin and thereby leads to intracellular trapping of iron ions and consequently to the development of an iron overload which resembles hereditary hemochromatosis. However, in contrast to hemochromatosis the central nervous system is also affected. Due to the impaired transferrin binding, however, iron concentrations and transferrin saturation in plasma are low whereas ferritin concentrations are high reflecting the impaired iron distribution and release.

In the so-called-"African Dietary Iron Overload" the increased dietary iron intake from excessive consumption of beer home-brewed in steel drums was long considered the only cause of this iron overload disorder resembling hemochromatosis. However, a non-HLA-linked gene has now additionally been implicated which, as in hemochromatosis, may impair the protective mechanism in the mucosal cells.

Disturbances of Iron Distribution

Malignant neoplasias and chronic inflammations lead to a shortage of transport and active iron, with simultaneous overloading of the iron stores. When tumors are present, the disturbance of the iron distribution is further influenced by the increased iron requirement of the tumor tissue. These conditions, like manifest iron deficiency, are characterized by anemia, low iron levels and low transferrin saturation values. Genuine iron deficiency is distinguished by reduced ferritin and elevated transferrin concentrations (Table 2).

The elevated ferritin concentration in these cases is not representative of the body's total iron reserves, but indicates the redistribution to the iron-storing tissue. The low transferrin saturation distinguishes disturbances of iron distribution from genuine iron overload conditions.

In the presence of tumors, the disturbed iron distribution with increased release of iron-rich basic isoferritins into the blood plasma is accompanied by separate synthesis of mainly acidic iron-poor isoferritins. Only a small fraction of the acidic isoferritins is normally detected by commercially available immunoassay methods, but at very high concentrations they can lead to raised ferritin concentrations. The total ferritin concentration is therefore underestimated in the presence of tumors; what is recorded is mainly the redistribution of iron, and to a smaller extent the autochthonous tumor synthesis products.

A non-representative elevation of the plasma ferritin concentration is also found in patients with cell necrosis of the iron-storage organs, e.g. in liver diseases.

In most of the iron distribution disturbances, there is a relative shortage in the amount of iron supplied to the erythropoietic cells, together with reduced erythropoietic activity. Correspondingly, transferrin receptor expression is usually normal. In the case of rapidly growing tumors, it can also be elevated as a result of the increased iron requirement of the tumor cells.

A very rare hereditary form of iron redistribution is caused by atransferrinemia. The lack of transferrin-bound iron transport leads to low iron concentrations in plasma and a reduced supply of all iron consuming cells. The transport function is taken over nonspecifically by other proteins such as albumin, leading to an uncontrolled deposition of iron in cells, which is not regulated according to demand by transferrin receptor expression.

Anemias of Chronic Diseases (ACD) in Inflammations

As described above, iron redistribution with a relative over-loading of iron stores and concomitant relative iron deficiency of erythropoietic cells (as a consequence of reduced transferrin synthesis) can occur mainly in chronic inflammation and also in tumors. This represents a major pathomechanism of the development of anemias of infection and malignancy. If the redistribution of iron is predominant, then hypochromic anemia is highly probable and can be differentiated from iron deficiency anemia by ferritin assays.

Apart from down-regulation of transferrin, a second cause of iron redistribution in inflammations has recently been identified [18, 45, 141, 142]. Increased production of cytokines IFN-γ and TNF-α stimulates iron uptake in macrophages by increased transferrin receptor expression. As a consequence, increased iron uptake induces increased ferritin synthesis, which in turn causes enhanced ferritin release into plasma. Increased iron storage in macrophages in ACD draws iron from transferrin; in contrast to true iron overload, this kind of iron redistribution is characterized by a low transferrin saturation. Cytokine induced iron uptake is mediated by nitric oxide (NO). Iron redistribution inhibits growth of tumor cells and microorganisms and may also enhance cytokine effects (Fig. 15), whereas iron availability for Hb synthesis is reduced [142].

Iron Redistribution in ACD

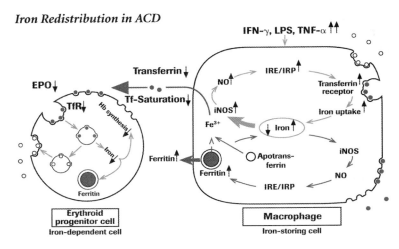

Fig. 15. Model of the autoregulatory loop between iron metabolism and the NO/NOS pathway in activated monocytes/macrophages and supply of an iron dependent cell. [141, 142]

Abbreviations: IFN-γ, interferon γ; iNOS = inducible nitric oxide synthase; IRE, iron-responsive element; IRE/IRP high-affinity binding of iron-regulatory protein (IRP) to IREs; LPS, lipopolysaccharide; TNF-α, tumor necrosis factor α; ↑ and ↓ indicate increase or decrease of cellular responses, respectively.

Explanation of signs:

         ⌒ transferrin receptor,   ● iron-carrying transferrin,

         O apotransferrin,   ◎ ferritin.

Iron stored as ferritin within an iron-storing cell is released and bound to apotransferrin, and then carried to the iron-requiring cell. The cytoplasmic membrane contains transferrin receptors to which the iron-carrying transferrin binds. The endosome migrates into the cytoplasm where it releases iron. The free iron is either used as functional iron or is stored as ferritin. The endosome returns to the cytoplasmic membrane and apotransferrin is released into the extracellular space.

This vicious circle can possibly be broken by substitution of erythropoietin and iron, which stimulates erythropoiesis and iron uptake by bone marrow cells and conversely draws iron from macrophages, thereby reducing cytotoxic effects.

Another cause of ACD results from reduced erythropoiesis activity which is due to an inadequate erythropoietin response to anemia and tissue hypoxia [45, 90, 101]. In contrast to renal anemia this is not an erythropoietin deficiency but rather a cytokine determined dysregulation. This means that the anemia cannot be compensated by increased erythropoietin synthesis, furthermore erythropoetin effects are reduced.

In certain cases a hemolytic component also contributes to pathogenesis of anemia, for example due to autoantibodies in the context of a malignant systemic disease or an autoimmune disease.

If hemolysis or a reduced erythropoietin response is the predominant factor in the genesis of the ACD, then the anemia may be normocytic in character rather than microcytic. In the case of marked hemolysis the reticulocyte count is in the normal to elevated range. If, in contrast, iron redistribution and diminished erythropoietic activity is predominant then a lowered reticulocyte count and microcytic anemia is to be expected.

Anemias of Malignancy

The mechanisms responsible for anemia of chronic disease in inflammations described above, such as downregulation of transferrin production, iron redistribution into macrophages as well as an insufficient erythropoietin response are also defective in tumor anemia and fulfill an urgent biological purpose since tumor cells are hereby iron depleted and growth-inhibited.

Furthermore, in malignant diseases of the hematopoietic system induction of autoantibodies and splenomegaly may contribute to increased hemolysis which as a long-term effect leads to an iron overload in addition to iron redistribution.

In all malignant diseases with significant bone marrow infiltration not only erythropoiesis but hematopoiesis in general may be reduced. This is the prognostically most unfavorable form of a tumor anemia with respect to responsiveness to substitution of iron and erythropoietin. This is also true for myelodysplastic syndromes in which an increased but ineffective erythropoiesis is characterized by a maximal stimulation of erythropoietin production which finally also leads to an iron overload state. These bone marrow diseases can only be diagnosed adequately by bone marrow investigation by hematologically experienced experts. Furthermore, tumor-associated hemorrhage may aggravate the anemia and, if marked, lead to iron depletion in contrast to the situation described above.

Disturbances of Iron Utilization

Even with normal iron reserves and normal iron distribution, indicated by a normal serum ferritin concentration, disturbances of iron utilization or incorporation possibly simulate the presence of iron-deficiency anemia as they also lead to microcytic or normocytic anemia. Ever since erythropoietin has replaced the transfusions previously used to treat renal anemia, dialysis patients have constituted the largest group. Despite adequate iron reserves, under erythropoietin therapy it is not always possible to mobilize sufficient iron from the iron stores, a situation which is shown, for example, as a reduction in transport iron (low transferritin saturation). Similarly, as in genuine iron deficiency and disturbances of iron distribution induced by tumors or infections, the reduced availability of iron in heme synthesis leads to compensation by increased incorporation of zinc into the porphyrin ring. This can be measured as increased Zn-protoporphyrin in the erythrocytes, and can be used as an additional aid to the diagnosis of iron utilization disturbances with normal or elevated ferritin concentrations. However, the iron-storage protein ferritin is the only suitable means of distinguishing between genuine iron deficiency and disturbances of iron distribution or utilization, whereas transferrin saturation is considered the best indicator of mobilized iron.

Rare forms of sideroachrestic anemias are caused by MDS (Myelodis plastic Syndrome), vitamin B_6 deficiency, lead intoxication or erythropoietic porphyrias (see „Disturbances of Porphyrin Synthesis").

Renal Anemias

Particular attention should also be paid to iron metabolism in patients with renal anemia. The substitution of erythropoietin, together with the i.v. administration of iron, has replaced transfusions which used to be performed routinely, and has therefore revolutionized therapy.

While previously regular transfusions, with the concomitant disturbance of iron utilization due to erythropoietin deficiency, almost invariably led to increasing iron overload, with all the associated consequences, the disturbances of iron metabolism in dialysis patients are now fundamentally different: usually the iron reserves are adequate, i.e. the ferritin concentration is normal, or possibly increased if earlier transfusions or even iron replacement treatment have been carried out.

Despite normal iron reserves, iron mobilization is typically disturbed, which is indicated by low transferrin saturation, which can lead to relative short supply of iron in erythropoiesis and to so-called functional iron deficiency. Generally this situation cannot be remedied by oral iron replacement therapy as, in most cases, iron absorption is also disturbed. However, as long as the erythropoietin deficiency typical of renal anemia is not corrected, the erythropoietic activity is reduced to the same extent as the iron mobilization. Therefore at a low level, iron turnover and erythropoiesis are in a steady state, which is then manifested in low transferrin receptor expression.

Renal anemia can also be complicated by a hemolytic component as a result of mechanical damage of the red cells during hemodialysis. If this is the case, a normal or even elevated reticulocyte count is to be expected as a compensatory mechanism.

However, if attempts are made to correct the erythropoietin deficiency by replacement, thereby increasing erythropoietic activity, the poor mobilization of the iron reserves is apparent as a functional iron deficiency. The cells of erythropoiesis react by increased expression of the transferrin receptor to improve iron provision. Further studies still have to be carried out on the extent to which the concentration of the soluble transferrin receptor correctly reflects the iron requirement of erythropoiesis in this case. Until now, the already well-established parameters of iron metabolism have formed the basis for the assessment. The ferritin concentration is generally a true reflection of the iron reserves (an exception to this is when it is immediately preceded by iron replacement or in the presence of a secondary disorder involving iron distribution disturbances) and can therefore be used as a guideline for recognizing any depot iron deficiency or for avoiding iron overload in iron replacement therapy. Transferrin saturation is currently the best indicator of the presence of mobilized transport iron and is inversely proportional to the iron requirement. Reduced transferrin saturation in dialysis patients is a sign of inadequate iron mobilization and therefore of a functional iron deficiency requiring iron replacement. It may be possible in the future to use the concentration of the soluble transferrin receptor as a direct indicator of the iron requirement. However, because of the lack of Standardisation generally valid decision criteria can not be given yet. On no account can the transferrin receptor replace the ferritin determination for assesing the iron reserves as it only reflects the current erythropoietic activity and/or its iron requirement, which do not necessarily correlate with the iron reserves. Determination of the zinc protoporphyrin in the erythrocytes has no advantage over the parameters mentioned. Because of the 120-day life-span of the erythrocytes, this determination would only reflect the iron metabolism situation at too late a stage (Table 3) [57].

Pathophysiology of Erythropoietin Production

Renal anemia is the prime example of true erythropoietin deficiency [35, 36]. In progressive renal disease, erythropoietin producing cells in peritubulary capillaries lose their production

Table 3. Estimation of iron metabolism in dialysis patients

Iron reserves	Transport iron
Ferritin	*Transferrin saturation*
Generally adequate or elevated (due to transfusions, Fe replacement, disturbed Fe mobilization)	Currently best indicator for mobilizable iron
Iron absorption	Iron requirement
(Fe absorption test)	Inversely proportional to transferrin saturation
Generally abnormal, therefore i.v. Fe administration if required	(zinc protoporphyrin) soluble transferrin receptor

capacity leading to a breakdown of the autoregulatory loop which normally guarantees a constant hemoglobin concentration. In patients with renal disease this, together with disturbed iron mobilization, can usually be assumed to be the cause of the anemia. Confirmation by determination of erythropoietin is only necessary in doubtful cases. On the other hand, an insufficient erythropoietin response, probably due to cytokine effects, is probably one of the major causes of anemia of chronic disease (ACD) apart from iron redistribution. Absolute erythropoietin concentrations are frequently found to be within the reference range for clinically healthy persons, however this can be considered to be inadequate in patients with anemia. This state can only be interpreted correctly if measured erythropoietin levels are related to the blood count. Inadequate erythropoietin secretion and efficacy and the corresponding iron redistribution can, however, be corrected by erythropoietin and iron therapy, as in renal anemia.

In contrast to these diseases caused by erythropoietin deficiency or insufficient response, all other anemias lead to an increased erythropoietin production as a measure of compensation. This is true for very different causes of anemia, for instance iron deficiency anemia, hemolytic anemias and many bone marrow diseases with inefficient erythropoiesis. In severe bone marrow damage (for instance aplastic anemia, myelodysplasia) this compensatory mechanism is not effective anymore because the erythroid progenitor cells are missing or fail to mature.

Increased erythropoietin secretion which is not a compensation for anemia may lead to a secondary erythrocytosis, provided a sufficient iron supply and normal bone marrow function are present. In hypoxia (cardiopulmonary diseases, heavy smokers, high altitude, athletes) this is a mechanism of adaptation to oxygen deficiency. In rare cases, however, carcinomas of the kidney or the liver may produce erythropoietin which also leads to erythrocytosis [65]. In contrast to these secondary forms of erythrocytosis, polycythemia vera is an autonomous proliferation of erythroid cells which leads to a compensatory down-regulation of erythropoietin production. Determination of erythropoietin can therefore contribute to the differential diagnosis of erythrocytosis in doubtful cases.

Non-iron-induced Disturbances of Erythropoiesis

Disturbances of Stem Cell Proliferation

Even at stem-cell level, physiological cell maturation can be compromised by numerous noxae and deficiencies, which in this case leads not only to anemia, but also to disturbances of myelopoiesis and thrombocytopoiesis. Examples that can be cited are medullary aplasia induced by autoimmune (e.g. thymoma), infectious (e.g., hepatitis) or toxic (e.g., antineoplastic drugs, benzene) processes or ionizing radiation. Chemical noxae or irradiation can, however, also lead to hyperregenerative bone-marrow insufficiency (myelodysplasia) with iron overload and a possible transition to acute leukemia. Whereas the above-mentioned diseases can be adequately diagnosed only by invasive and costly bone-marrow investigations, the causes of vitamin-deficiency-induced disturbances of the proliferation and maturation of bone-marrow cells with macrocytic anemia can be

Disturbances of Iron Utilization 41

Table 4. EPO and ferritin concentrations in anemias and erythrocytosis

Disease	EPO concentration	Ferritin concentration
Anemias		
Iron deficiency	↑	↓
Renal anemia	↓–↓↓	n-↑
Anemia of chronic disease	n-↓	n-↑↑
Hemolysis	↑	n-↑
Bone marrow diseases with ineffective erythropoiesis	↑	↑–↑↑
Erythrocytosis		
Reactive in hypoxia	↑	variable
Paraneoplastic (e.g., kidney, liver carcinoma)	↑↑	n-↑
Polycythemia vera	n-↓	n-↑

detected more simply by the determination of vitamin B_{12} or folic acid in the serum. However, the differentiation of MDS and vitamin B_{12} and folic acid deficiency may be difficult due to similar megaloblastic alterations in bone marrow and macrocytic anemia in all these cases.

Vitamin B_{12} and Folic Acid Deficiency

Since the very low daily cobalamin requirement of about 2 μg can be easily covered with a normal, varied diet, diet-induced vitamin B_{12} deficiency is rare, except in radical vegetarians. The vast majority of deficiency syndromes are therefore caused either by a deficiency of intrinsic factor (chronic atrophic gastritis, gastric resection, antibodies to intrinsic factor) or by disturbances of absorption (fish tapeworm, intestinal diseases). By contrast, folic acid deficiency arises mainly as a result of unbalanced diet and reduced storage in liver damage, especially in connection with alcoholism. Other important causes are malabsorption in intestinal diseases and inhibition of the folic acid synthesis of intestinal bacteria by antibacterial or cytotoxic chemotherapy with folic acid antagonists. The intracellular bioavailability of the active form tetrahydrofolic acid also depends on an adequate supply of vitamin C (reduction) and in particular of vitamin B_{12} (intracellular uptake and demethylation). Since, for this reason and on account of the transfer of C_1 units, folic acid and vitamin B_{12} act synergistically in DNA synthesis and cell maturation, deficiencies similarly lead to macrocytic anemia. On account of the reduced proliferation capacity, especially of the cells of erythropoiesis, the total count of erythrocytes is then significantly reduced. However since the hemoglobin synthesis capacity is at the same time normal, the individual erythrocytes are not only abnormally large ("macrocytes", Fig. 17) but also have an elevated hemoglobin content ("hyperchromic anemia"). In view of the fact that the forms of anemia are the same and that folic acid is active only with an adequate vitamin B_{12} supply, a first diagnosis of macrocytic anemia requires the simultaneous determination of vitamin B_{12} and folic acid and possibly the exclusion of MDS.

If folic acid deficiency is suspected, then the serum folic acid concentration may be within the lower reference range. This can indicate a latent folic acid deficiency which can possibly be proven by determining the folic acid content of erythrocytes or homocysteine [15]. If serum concentrations are normal but the erythrocytes are nevertheless supplied with an insufficient amount of folic acid then an uptake disorder is manifest which is most often caused by a vitamin B_{12} deficiency.

As a result of new findings, latent vitamin B_{12} or folic acid deficiency have recently also received more attention. Manifestations of this latent vitamin deficiency prior to the appearance of anemia or funicular spinal disease in vitamin B_{12} deficiency can lead to other metabolic anomalies such as hyperhomocysteinemia, an elevated risk of neural tube defects, immune deficiencies and atherosclerosis. (Fig. 16)

Recently the term "metabolic vitamin B_{12} or folic acid deficiency" has been introduced. It is characterized by the presence of deficiency symptoms (predominantly macrocytic anemia) already at vitamin B_{12} or folic acid concentrations in the lower reference range, possibly due to an increased demand sometimes in

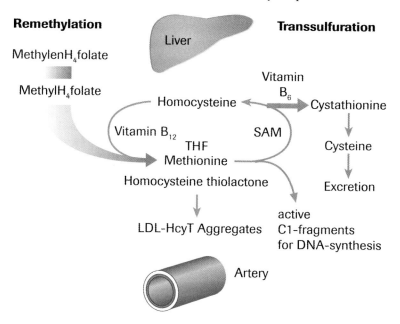

Fig. 16. Metabolism of homocysteine, folate, vitamin B12, vitamin B6 according to Herrmann W et al. Clin Lab 1997; 43: 1005-9.

     SAM: S-Adenosyl-Methionin

     THF: Tetrahydrofolate

     LDL-HycT Aggregates: Low-Density-Lipoprotein-Homocystein-Transferase-Aggregates

the context of MDS or neoplasia. This may be confirmed by further laboratory investigations. Latent or functional folic acid deficiency leads to hyperhomocysteinemia, latent and functional vitamin B_{12} deficiency mainly to an increased concentration of methylmalonic acid and possibly also of homocysteine. Vitamin B_{12} deficiency can be considered very unlikely, however, if the serum concentration is above 300 ng/l. This is also true for folic acid concentrations within a functionally defined reference range above 4.4 ng/ml.

Hemoglobinopathies

Hemoglobinopathies are a disturbance in the synthesis of the protein components of hemoglobin [28]. A distinction is made between point mutations with exchange of individual amino acids and defects in whole protein chains. Of the former, sickle-cell anemia is the most important because it is widespread in the black population of Africa and America. The substitution of valine for glutaminic acid as sixth amino acid in the β-chain leads to the synthesis of so-called sickle-cell hemoglobin (HbS) which has a very low solubility when it is not O_2 saturated. In oxygen deficiency, the change in conformation leads to precipitation of the HbS and the appearance of the characteristic sickle-shaped red cells (drepanocytes, Fig. 17). These are visible under the microscope and can therefore be used diagnostically. Atypical sick-

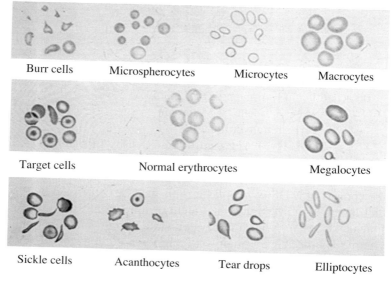

| Burr cells | Microspherocytes | Microcytes | Macrocytes |

| Target cells | Normal erythrocytes | Megalocytes |

| Sickle cells | Acanthocytes | Tear drops | Elliptocytes |

Fig. 17. Normal and pathological forms of erythrocytes modified by Diem H [Begemann H, Rastetter J (1987) Atlas der klinischen Hämatologie, 4. Aufl. Springer, Berlin Heidelberg New York Tokyo]

le-cell hemoglobin can also be detected by hemoglobin electrophoresis.

Hemoglobinopathies in the broader sense also include the so-called thalassemias. The widespread immigration into Central and Northern Europe from the Mediterranean area, has greatly increased the importance of these disorders, especially in pediatrics. The term refers to a condition in which there is reduced synthesis or complete absence of entire chains from the hemoglobin molecule. Since α-chains are contained in fetal HbF as well as in HbA_0 and HBA_2, α-chain thalassemia has an impact on the fetus and patients of all ages. The absence of the α-chains is offset in the fetus by the formation of tetramers from γ-chains ($Hb\gamma_4$ = Bart's Hb), after birth by the formation of tetramers from β-chains ($Hb\beta_4$ = Hb H). Erythrocytes with these pathological hemoglobins have a tendency to aggregate, however, and are broken down early. Since the synthesis of α-chains is coded for by 4 genes, 4 clinical pictures of varying severity can be identified, depending on the number of defective genes: a defect in one gene is manifested merely as an increased proportion of the above-mentioned pathological variants of hemoglobin, a 2-gene defect produces mild, a 3-gene defect pronounced anemia with premature hemolysis. The complete loss of the α-chains is incompatible with the survival of the fetus.

By contrast with α-thalassemia, β-thalassemia does not have an effect until infancy or childhood when the γ-chains are replaced by β-chains. If this is not possible, HbF (with γ-chains) and HbA_2 (with δ-chains) is formed by way of compensation. Depending on its mode of inheritance, a distinction can be made between a heterozygous form (thalassemia minor) with reduced β-chain synthesis and correspondingly milder anemia, and a homozygous form (thalassemia major) with more or less complete absence of β-chains and severe anemia.

The pathological variants of hemoglobin in thalassemia lead to characteristic abnormalities in the shape of erythrocytes (microcytic anemia with target cells, Fig. 17), which are detectable microscopically, whereas more precise differentiation is possible only by hemoglobin electrophoresis.

Pathophysiologically, these structural and morphological abnormalities of erythrocytes result in more or less pronounced insufficiency as oxygen carriers and lead to an increased aggregation tendency. In addition, deformation also leads to accelerated destruction of erythrocytes, predominantly in the spleen, with all the signs of corpuscular hemolytic anemia. For signs of hemolysis and hemolytically-determined iron overload, see under "Pathologically Increased Hemolysis".

Disturbances of Porphyrin Synthesis

Disturbances of prophyrin synthesis [26] are to be considered here only in so far as they may affect erythropoiesis and lead to anemia (Fig. 18).

These forms of anemia are called sideroachrestic, since the iron provided for Hb synthesis in the bone marrow cannot be used, despite adequate reserves, and is consequently stored in the erythroblasts. The erythroblasts, which are thus overloaded with iron, are then termed sideroblasts, and can be detected in the bone marrow using iron-specific stains. In sideroachrestic anemia, however, the inadequately increased iron absorption results in the development of generalized, genuine iron overload over a longer period, but especially after repeated transfusions; it is recognizable from an elevated serum ferritin concentration. Most of the causes of sideroachrestic anemia are comparatively uncommon, and therefore rarely need to be considered in practice. Hereditary erythropoietic porphyrias such as congenital erythropoietic uroporphyria (Günther's disease) with a defect of uroporphyrinogen III synthase and erythropoietic protoporphyria with a defect of ferrochelatase are particularly rare. Acquired forms such as pyridoxal phosphate (vitamin B_6) deficiency are slightly more common; this may be of nutritional origin, in alcoholics, for example, or arise as a result of isoniazid therapy in tuberculosis patients, and leads to a disturbance of iron incorporation via inhibition of δ-amino-levulinic acid synthase and

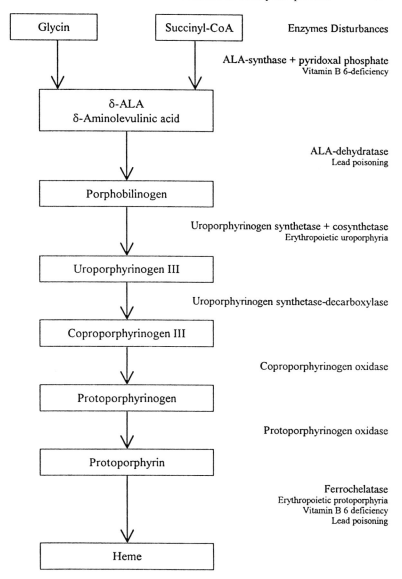

Fig. 18. Disturbances of prophyrin synthesis with possible anemia

ferrochelatase. Similar pathological mechanisms are also at the root of lead-induced anemia and disturbance of porphyrin synthesis. Chronic lead intoxication leads to inhibition of δ-aminolevulinic acid dehydratase and of ferrochelatase. All the above-mentioned causes ultimately produce a disturbance of iron utilization via the synthesis of an incomplete porphyrin skeleton or via the direct inhibition of ferrochelatase, with the general features of sideroachrestic (sideroblastic) anemia described above. If the defect is mainly in the terminal stage of the reaction (incorporation of iron by ferrochelatase), zinc is incorporated into the finished protoporphyrin skeleton instead of iron, recognizable from the increased concentration of Zn-protoporphyrin in the erythrocytes. Defects at earlier stages in porphyrin synthesis can be identified by analysis of the corresponding intermediate products; lead and vitamin B_6 can also be determined directly for confirmation of the diagnosis.

Pathologically Increased Hemolysis

„Hemolysis" is the term generally used in clinical medicine to describe the pathologically increased or premature destruction of erythrocytes. The cause of this may lie in structural or biochemical defects in the erythrocytes themselves ("corpuscular hemolysis"), in which case it takes place mainly in the macrophages of the RES in the spleen or the liver. By contrast, extracorpuscular hemolysis takes place mainly intravascularly through the action of autoantibodies, toxins, infective organisms or physical noxae, such as artificial heart valves. Intravascular hemolysis can be detected very sensitively by means of clinico-chemical investigations, since hemoglobin and erythrocyte enzymes, e.g. LDH isoenzymes 1 and 2, pass into the peripheral blood even at a low hemolysis rate.

Haptoglobin

Since free hemoglobin is rapidly bound to α_2-haptoglobin and this hemoglobin-haptoglobin complex is also rapidly phagocytized by the RES, a selective reduction in free haptoglobin is regarded as the most sensitive sign of intravascular hemolysis which at the same time also has a high degree of diagnostic specificity [95]. The only other possible causes are severe protein-loss syndromes or disturbances of protein synthesis. This applies in particular to advanced liver diseases (e.g. liver cirrhosis) with a severe synthesis defect which also includes haptoglobin. A reduction in haptoglobin may also be produced, albeit less commonly, by gastrointestinal protein-loss syndromes which also non-selectively include macromolecular proteins, such as celiac disease, Whipple's disease. Since haptoglobin also serves as a proteinase inhibitor, its synthesis in the liver is increased during acute-phase reactions. The resultant increase in concentration may then "mask" any hemolysis which is present simultaneously (Table 5).

Features of Severe Hemolysis

Free hemoglobin occurs in the plasma only if the hemoglobin binding capacity of haptpoglobin is exceeded; if the renal threshold is exceeded, excretion in the urine is also possible. Excess heme can also be bound in the blood by hemopexin and be removed from the plasma in the form of a heme-hemopexin complex. Hemoglobinuria and a reduction in serum hemopexin are thus signs of severe hemolysis. The degradation of heme leads,

Table 5. Differentiation: Hemolysis, acute-phase reaction and protein loss or disturbance of protein synthesis

Disease	Haptoglobin	Hemopexin	CRP
Mild hemolysis	↓-↓↓	n	n
Severe hemolysis	↓↓	↓	n
Hemolysis and acute-phase reaction	n-↑	n-↓	↑↑
Acute-phase reaction	↑-↑↑	n	↑↑
Nephrotic syndrome	↑-↑↑	↓	n-↓
Gastrointestinal protein loss or disturbance of protein synthesis	↓	↓	n-↓

independently of the site of the hemolytic process, to an increased amount of unconjugated bilirubin and of iron. Because of the simultaneous inappropriately increased iron absorption and the possible need for transfusions, all chronic forms of hemolysis are associated with iron overload, recognizable as an increased serum ferritin concentration. With adequate bone marrow function, increased hemolysis, especially extracorpuscular forms, can be compensated for by new formation which can be boosted up to 10-fold. This is shown as an increased passage of immature erythrocytes (reticulocytes) into the peripheral blood. Anemia develops only if the hemolysis rate exceeds the bone marrow capacity.

If, in the long run, the binding capacity of haptoglobin and hemopexin is exceeded during severe intravascular hemolysis and as a consequence of this larger amounts of free hemoglobin are filtered through the glomeruli and therefore excreted, then in individual cases because of the chronic loss of iron, the hemolysis may lead to iron deficiency. If, however, iron loss does not occur in this manner, then iron overload is usually the consequence of chronic hemolysis as described above. This can be differentiated by regular urine investigations and ferritin determinations in serum.

Causes of Hemolysis

Corpuscular Hemolysis

Corpuscular hemolysis can also be induced by defects in the erythrocyte membrane, in addition to the hemoglobinopathies such as sickle-cell anemia or thalassemia mentioned earlier. The most important example of such a membrane defect is spherocytic anemia (hereditary spherocytosis) which can be diagnosed on the basis of the characteristic morphological changes ("spherocytes") (Table 6) and the reduced osmotic resistance of the erythrocytes. Other causes are defects of erythrocyte enzymes which are required for the stabilization of functionally important proteins, e.g. glucose-6-phosphatedehydrogenase deficiency. Whereas this disease has also become

Table 6. Diagnosis of corpuscular hemolytic anemias

Disease	Erythrocyte forms	Confirmation test
Hereditary spherocytosis	Microspherocytes	Osmotic resistance
Thalassemia	Target cells	Hemoglobin electrophoresis, PCR
Sickle cell anemia	Sickle cells	Hemoglobin electrophoresis, PCR
Erythrocyte enzyme defects (e.g. Gluc-6-PD-deficiency)	unspecific Heinz Bodies	Erythrocyte enzymes
PNH (paroxysmal nocturnal hemoglobinuria or Marchiafava-Micheli Syndrome)	unspecific	Defect of glycolipid anchor antigens such as CD59 and CD55

important in Central and Northern Europe as a result of immigration from the Mediterranean area, all other defects of erythrocyte enzymes are definitely rarities.

Extracorpuscular Hemolysis

Numerous noxae, most of which can be identified from the case history or by means of simple laboratory investigations, produce intravascular hemolysis by directly damaging the erythrocytes themselves; these include mechanical hemolysis after heart valve replacement, toxins such as snake venoms or detergents, and infective organisms such as malarial plasmodia, or hemolysis as a consequence of gram-negative sepsis. Intravascular hemolysis can be identified independently of the causes on the basis of the above-mentioned general features of hemolysis. However, in the case of the autoimmune hemolytic anemias which can occur in the context of autoimmune diseases, immune defects, viral infections, lymphatic malignancies and as drug-induced anemias, the causes are often difficult to determine in the individual case. A distinction is made between so-called warm, cold and bithermal (Donath-Landsteiner) antibodies; binding of the antibodies to the patient's erythrocytes can be detected in the direct anti-human globulin test (Coombs' test) and, if the result is positive, further differentiation using other methods is necessary.

Diagnosis of Disturbances of Iron Metabolism
Disturbances of Erythropoiesis

Knowledge of physiological principles and the acquisition of clinical laboratory data are tools used by the doctor in clinical practice. However, it is becoming increasingly difficult to interpret the mass of data from the clinical laboratory and to correlate the findings with the patient's clinical status.

How should the laboratory results be interpreted to enable the clinician to act on them more quickly and efficiently?

The Body's Iron Balance

The iron balance is controlled entirely by absorption. The uptake of iron therefore occupies the key position in the iron metabolism as a whole (Fig. 19).

The daily iron requirement depends on age and sex. It is increased in puberty and in pregnancy. Under physiological conditions, the total iron pool is more or less constant in adults. The quantity of iron absorbed is about 10% (1 mg) of the quantity consumed daily in the normal diet, but this fraction can increase to 20 to 40% (2 to 4 mg) in conditions of iron deficiency.

Physiological loss of iron is low, and comparable to the quantity absorbed. It takes place as a result of the shedding of intestinal epithelial cells and through excretion in bile, urine and perspiration. Since the absorption and the loss of iron are limited under physiological conditions, the quantity of storage iron can only be increased by massive supplies from outside the body.

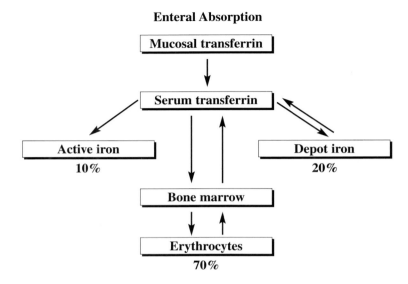

Fig. 19. Utilization of iron

Thus, every transfusion of one liter of blood increases the quantity of storage iron in the body by about 250 mg. A prolonged increased intake of iron also increases this quantity, unless there is a compensating blood loss, e.g. via the gastrointestinal tract.

Disturbances in iron absorption can be detected by an iron absorption test. This is of particular interest in iron deficiency of unknown origin and to demonstrate excessive iron absorption in primary hemochromatosis.

Iron Absorption Test

The iron absorption test should be carried out as follows:
- The blood sample should be collected from a fasting patient to determine the baseline value for the serum iron concentration.
- Oral administration of a bivalent iron preparation (200 mg Fe^{++}).
- A second blood collection after 3 hours.
- Alternatively, when there is a definite suspicion of disturbed absorption kinetics: blood collection after 1, 2, 3, 4 and 5 hours.

Interpretation of the iron absorption test: With normal iron absorption, there should be an increase to 2-3 times the baseline value during the observation period. A reduced or delayed rise indicates secondary iron overload or a disturbance of iron absorption which may result in an iron deficiency. By contrast, an accelerated or increased rise is found in forms of iron deficiency which are not due to a disturbance of absorption, and in primary hemochromatosis [144].

The iron balance is held constant ± 1 to 2 mg per day, and is regulated via the absorption capacity of the intestinal mucosa. The body generally stores enough iron to compensate for sudden extreme blood losses. The excess that is not used for the synthesis of hemoglobin, myoglobin, or iron enzymes is stored in the depot proteins ferritin and hemosiderin.

The total iron content of the healthy human body is about 3.5 to 4 g in women and 4 to 5 g in men [89]. About 70% of this is stored in hemoglobin, 10% is contained in iron-containing enzymes and myoglobin, 20% in the body's iron depot, and only 0.1 to 0.2% is bound to transferrin as transport iron. However, this distribution applies only under optimum nutritional conditions (Fig. 20).

Hemoglobin accounts for approximately 85% of the active iron. An iron content of 3.4 mg is calculated per gram of hemoglobin. Since the life cycle of the red blood cells is 120 days, an adult requires about 16 to 20 mg of iron daily in order to replace these vital cells [13]. Most of the iron required for this purpose comes from lysed red blood cells.

During pregnancy, birth, and breast-feeding, the additional iron requirement is far in excess of the quantity of absorbable iron contained in the food. The loss of iron in normal menstruation is about 15 to 30 mg (100 ml of blood contains about 50 mg of iron). The additional iron requirement during pregnancy is between 700 and 1000 mg.

The second largest component in active iron is myoglobin, at about 10%. Like hemoglobin, myoglobin is an oxygen-binding hemoprotein with a molecular weight of about 17,100 daltons. It

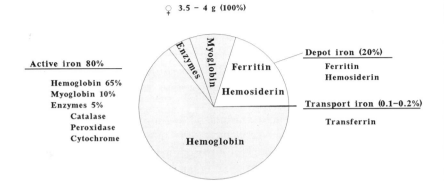

Fig. 20. Total content of iron in the body

is formed in the striated muscle (skeletal muscle and myocardium). Because it has a higher affinity for oxygen than hemoglobin, myoglobin is responsible for the transportation and storage of oxygen in the striated muscles.

The diagnostic specificity of the serum myoglobin determination is limited, since it is not possible to differentiate between skeletal muscle myoglobin and myocardium myoglobin. An increase in the serum is observed in all forms of muscle disease and injuries, and in myocardial infarction. The diagnostic value in the assessment of impaired kidney function is limited, since myoglobin is degraded to monomers and is completely eliminated with the urine. The determination of myoglobin in sports medicine for the assessment of performance is worthy of mention.

As a result of menstruation and pregnancy, the quantity of depot iron in women decreases through blood loss to 250 mg, i.e. only 5 to 10% of the total iron content. According to a WHO estimate, 50% of all fertile women in western countries suffer from hypoferremia.

Table 7. Distribution of iron in the human body

		♂ 70 kg		♀ 60 kg	
		mg	%	mg	%
Active iron	Hemoglobin	2800	66	2500	70
	Myoglobin	200	4	150	4
	Enzymes	400	10	350	10
Transport iron	Transferrin	4	0.1	4	0.1
Depot iron	Ferritin	800	20	500	16
	Hemosiderin				
Σ ~		4200	100	3500	100

Clinical Significance of the Determination of Ferritin

Massive disturbances of the iron balance can be detected by measurement of the body's iron stores (deficiency or overload). Disturbances of the distribution of iron between active iron, storage iron, and transport iron are also observed. The ferritin concentration reflects the total body iron stores. Additional indices (transferrin, transferrin saturation, and hematological investigations) are required for the diagnosis of disturbances of distribution.

Ferritin is the most important iron storage protein. Together with the quantitatively and biologically less important hemosiderin, it contains about 15 to 20% of all the iron in the body. Ferritin occurs in nearly all organs. Particularly high concentrations are found in liver, spleen, and bone marrow.

A direct correlation is found for healthy adults between the plasma ferritin concentration and the quantity of available iron stored in the body. Comparative studies with quantitative phlebotomies and the histochemical assessment of bone marrow aspirates have shown that in iron deficiency and in primary or secondary stages of iron overload ferritin provides accurate information on the iron reserves available to the body for hemoglobin synthesis [68].

If more iron is supplied than the body can store as ferritin, iron is deposited as hemosiderin in the cells of the reticuloendothelial

Table 8. Merits of the various parameters for the
detection of iron deficiency (according to Mazza J,)

	Sensitivity in %	Specificity in %	Efficiency in %
Serum iron +	84	43	52
Transferrin	84	63	67
Serum ferritin	79	96	92
Serum iron +			
Serum ferritin	84	42	51
Transferrin +			
Serum ferritin	84	50	64

system. Unlike ferritin, hemosiderin is insoluble in water, and it is only with difficulty that its iron content can be mobilized.

The value of ferritin determination was demonstrated more than 10 years ago in a comparison of the various parameters available for the determination of the body's iron stores.

Ferritin is well suited for assessment of the iron metabolism of a patient population having no primary consumptive disease or chronic inflammation. The determination of ferritin is particularly useful in the diagnosis of disturbances of iron metabolism, in the monitoring of iron therapy, for the determination of iron reserves in high-risk groups, and in the differential diagnosis of anemias [83] (Tab. 9).

Representative Ferritin Levels – Size of Iron Stores

In clinical practice, the ferritin concentration reflects the size of the iron stores, especially at the beginning of therapy. A deficiency in the stores of the reticuloendothelial system (RES) can be detected at a particularly early stage. A value of 20 ng/ml has been found to be a suitable clinical limit for prelatent iron deficiency. A value below this reliably indicates exhaustion of the iron reserves that can be mobilized for hemoglobin synthesis. A decrease to less than 12 ng/ml is defined as latent iron deficiency. Neither of these values calls for further laboratory confirmation, even where the blood count is still morphologically

Table 9. Clinical significance of ferritin

1. Representative result
   Detection of prelatent and latent iron deficiency
   Differential diagnosis of anemias
   Monitoring of high-risk groups
   Monitoring of iron therapy (oral)
   Determination of the iron status of dialysis patients and patients who have
   received multiple blood transfusions
   Diagnosis of iron overload
   Monitoring of phlebotomy therapy or chelating agent therapy
2. Non-representative result
   Destruction of hepatocellular tissue
   Infections
   Inflammations (collagen diseases)
   Malignancies
   Iron therapy (parenteral)

Table 10. Ferritin concentrations in healthy individuals and in patients with iron deficiency and iron overload

	ng/ml = µg/l
Reference range	
– Men and women over 50 years of age	30-300
– Women under 50 years of age	10-160
Prelatent iron deficiency (storage iron deficiency)	< 20
Latent iron deficiency/iron deficiency anemia	< 12
Representative iron overload	> 400

normal. They are indications for therapy, though it is still necessary to look for the cause of the iron deficiency. If the reduced ferritin concentration is accompanied by hypochromic microcytic anemia, the patient is suffering from manifest iron deficiency.

If the ferritin level is elevated and a disturbance of distribution can be ruled out by determination of the transferrin saturation and/or of the C-reactive protein and by investigation of the blood sedimentation rate and the blood count, the raised ferritin level indicates that the body is overloaded with iron. A ferritin value of 400 ng/ml is taken as a limit. The transferrin saturation is massively increased (over 50%) in these cases.

If there is no evidence of any other disease, primary or secondary hemochromatosis must be suspected. Differential diagnosis must be pursued through history-taking, liver biopsy, bone-marrow puncture, or MRI. Diagnosis of a primary hemochromatosis calls for further investigations for organic lesions.

Transferrin, Transferrin Saturation

Raised non-representative ferritin values are ambiguous, and are found in a number of inflammatory diseases, in the presence of malignant growths, and in the presence of damage to the liver parenchyma. Elevated ferritin levels are also found in a number of anemias arising from various causes in some cases with true iron overload. Recent oral or, in particular, parenteral iron therapy can also lead to raised non-representative ferritin values.

These non-representative increases in the ferritin concentration are generally due to disturbances of distribution, and differential diagnosis is possible by determination of the transferrin concentration and of the transferrin saturation. In all these processes, the transferrin value is reduced or close to the lower limit of the reference range. The transferrin saturation is low to normal, and hypochromic anemia can often be diagnosed on the basis of the blood count.

Elevated transferrin values are found in the presence of iron deficiency and particularly in pregnancy. The transferrin level may also be raised as a result of drug induction (administration of oral contraceptives). A detailed patient history is essential.

A number of rare anemias with hyperferritinemia and low transferrin levels belong to the group of sideroachrestic diseases and are congenital hypochromic microcytic anemias (atransferrinemia, antitransferrin antibodies, receptor defects).

Increased ferritin concentrations together with low transferrin levels point to anemias with ineffective erythropoiesis (thalassemias, megaloblastic, sideroblastic, and dyserythropoietic anemias). Myelodysplastic syndromes, on the other hand, may be accompanied by elevated values for both transferrin and ferritin.

Table 11. Transferrin in the differential diagnosis of disturbances of iron metabolism

---

1. *Normal to slightly reduced transferrin concentrations*
   Primary hemochromatosis (exception: late stage secondary hemochromatosis)
2. *Decreased transferrin concentrations*
   Infections
   Inflammations/collagen diseases
   Malignant tumors
   Hemodialysis patients
   Cirrhosis of the liver – disturbances of synthesis
   Nephrotic syndrome – losses
   Ineffective erythropoiesis
   (e.g. sideroachrestic and megaloblastic anemias)
   Thalassemias
3. *Increased transferrin concentrations*
   Iron deficiency
   Estrogen-induced increase in synthesis (pregnancy, medication)
   Ineffective erythropoiesis (some forms, e. g. myelodysplastic syndromes)

Elevated ferritin concentrations unrelated to the iron stores are often found in patients with malignancies. Possible reasons that have been suggested for this phenomenon are increased ferritin synthesis by neoplastic cells, release of ferritin on decomposition of neoplastic tissue, and blockage of erythropoiesis as a result of chronic inflammatory processes in and around the tumor tissue. Ferritin determinations on patients with malignant tumors sometimes also record high concentrations of acidic isoferritins [83].

In the presence of inflammations, infectious diseases, or malignant tumors, low transferrin concentrations and low transferrin saturation values point to disturbances of iron distribution. Low transferrin concentrations may be caused either by losses (renal, intestinal) or by reduced synthesis (compensation, liver damage).

Low transferrin values found for patients with cirrhosis of the liver are usually due to the defective protein metabolism. In nephrotic syndrome, so much transferrin is lost via the urine that low transferrin levels are the rule. The excretion of transferrin in the urine is used to determine the selectivity of proteinuria. The transferrin concentration and the transferrin saturation are valuable aids in the differential diagnosis of raised ferritin concentrations. True iron overload is accompanied by increased transferrin saturation. Non-representative ferritin elevation in patients with disturbances of distribution is characterized by low transferrin saturation and low transferrin concentrations.

Transferrin Receptor

The presence and concentration level of the serum transferrin receptor are essentially determined by the iron status of the cells and by cell growth. In addition to determining ferritin and the erythropoietin activity, the determination of the circulating transferrin receptor was found to be a sensitive tool for establishing prelatent iron deficiency, for distinguishing iron deficiency due to the disturbance of iron utilization in chronic diseases and as a useful tool in determining iron deficiency during pregnancy [134]. Furthermore, its histochemical determination can indicate malignant or normal cell growth.

In uncomplicated iron deficiency, transferrin receptor is up-regulated to increase the iron supply in erythropoietic bone marrow cells. In contrast to that, ferritin production is low. These phenomena are detectable already at the stage of latent iron deficiency, i.e. preceding the development of a microcytic hypochromic anemia. As a rule, this is obvious by ferritin concentrations below 20 ng/ml alone however in doubtful cases the ratio between soluble transferrin receptor and ferritin may show this more clearly [106, 107, 130].

Since both these forms of anemia may present as hypochromic, microcytic anemia, further diagnostic measures are needed to distinguish true iron deficiency from iron redistribution in inflammations and tumors. Iron redistribution is characterized by an increase uptake of iron by macrophages, which in turn leads to a low transferrin saturation and thereby to a low availability of transport iron for hemoglobin production. Apart from insufficient erythropoietin response this is one of the major pathomechanisms in ACD, which in addition to the microcytic appearance may lead to a confusion with true iron deficiency. As a rule, both conditions can be distinguished by ferritin determination since only in true iron deficiency ferritin production is low, whereas iron redistribution leads to a usually increased ferritin production which in those cases is not representative anymore for the iron reserves. However, the decrease of ferritin in iron deficiency may be masked if iron deficiency is caused by bleeding tumors or inflammations which also leads to a kind of redistribution. In those cases, transferrin receptor is upregulated indicating the absolute iron deficiency while in uncomplicated ACD it is usually normal due to the concomitant decrease of iron supply and erythropoietic activity.

If however erythropoiesis in ACD is stimulated by erythropoietin therapy the state of low iron supply becomes manifest as a so-called functional iron deficiency. This in turn leads to an upregulation of transferrin receptor indicating an increasing iron demand. This is particularly true if a concomitant decrease of ferritin concentration below levels of 100 ng/ml is observed.

Renal anemia is characterized by a deficient erythropoietin production and consequently a very low erythropoietic activity reflected by a low transferrin receptor expression. Iron reserves are usually normal to increased, however mobilization of these and also intestinal absorption of iron are usually decreased, reflected by a low transferrin saturation. This iron mobilization disorder becomes manifest as a so-called functional iron deficiency if erythropoiesis is stimulated by erythropoietin substitution. This in turn leads to increased transferrin receptor expression indicating a higher demand of iron, particularly if transferrin saturation remains low and ferritin concentrations are falling, similarly to ACD.

In uncomplicated iron overload conditions, such as hereditary hemochromatosis or secondary hemosiderosis due to transfusions or iron supplementation the expression of transferrin receptor is regulated reciprocally to ferritin. However, this reaction is rather insensitive compared to the increase of ferritin, which reflects increasing storage iron. So ferritin, and in the case of hemochromatosis also transferrin saturation remain the most sensitive screening parameters for detection of iron overload and also for the assessment of the iron reserves. In uncomplicated cases 1 ng/ml serum ferritin can be expected to represent about 10 mg of iron reserves.

In hemolysis and some bone marrow diseases with increased, but ineffective erythropoiesis like MDS paradoxically a simultaneous increase of ferritin and soluble transferrin receptor may be found even in the absence of any therapy. This is due to the fact that erythropoietic progenitor cells in bone marrow are increased as a measure for compensation of anemia. This leads to an overexpression of transferrin receptor and, as a result of increased iron absorption or transfusions possibly also to an iron overload. In these cases increased sTfR does not indicate an increased iron need but only reflects increased erythropoietic activity which is associated with iron overload. In contrast to that states with bone marrow aplasia, f. i. aplastic anemia or patients undergoing bone marrow transplantation show low sTfR values due to the low number of erythropoietic progenitor cells able to response erythropoietin stimulation. In all these states, sTfR may be used to assist assessment of erythropoietic activity together with established parameters like reticulocyte count. However, this has to be investigated yet by further clinical studies.

Hemoglobin, reticulocyte count, ferritin and transferrin saturation are the established parameters to monitor the success and the iron needs during an iron and EPO therapy. Successful stimulation of erythropoiesis is shown by the so-called reticulocyte crisis, however an increase sTfR and a decrease in hypochromic erythrocytes may precede this. Ferritin and transferrin saturation are still the most important parameters to detect iron deficiency and avoid iron overload. However, in contrast to uncomplicated iron deficiency, iron redistribution and iron mobilization defects are usually considered to require iron substitution already in ferritin concentrations below 100 ng/ml. Apart from this so-called absolute iron deficiency, increased sTfR values at normal ferritin concentrations still show an increased iron demand. However, iron overload should be avoided and increased ferritin and transferrin saturation are now considered contraindications to iron substitution even in cases with increased transferrin receptor which then only represent increased erythropoietic activity.

Iron Deficiency and Decreased Ferritin Concentrations

In the case of a negative iron balance, the iron stores are reduced first; this can be seen from the measurement of ferritin. The (transferrin-bound) iron concentration decreases only at a relatively late stage (as shown by the lower transferrin saturation).

Diagnosis of non-manifest iron deficiency is practically impossible by clinical methods. The physical findings and the patient's subjective condition do not reveal any definitely attributable changes. The familiar clinical symptoms such as pallor, weakness, loss of concentration, exertional dyspnea, and reduced resistance to infection appear only with the development of anemia, i.e. after depletion of tissue iron has already taken place. The relatively specific changes in the skin and mucous membranes, atrophic glossitis and gastritis, cracks at the corners of the mouth, and atrophy of the hair and nails are late symptoms. An important observation is that iron deficiency very often accompanies serious, life-threatening conditions, and can therefore serve as an indicator of such diseases.

Only laboratory tests can confirm a diagnosis of iron deficiency and, depending on the pattern of the results, it is possible to distinguish between prelatent, latent, and manifest iron deficiencies. In prelatent iron deficiency, the body's iron reserves are reduced. Latent iron deficiency is characterized by a reduced supply of iron for erythropoiesis. This gives way to manifest iron deficiency, which is characterized by typical iron deficiency anemia (Table 12).

Table 12. Iron status

	DEFICIENCY			OVERLOAD	
	Prelatent	Latent	Manifest	Primary	Secondary
Ferritin (ng/ml)	< 20	< 12	< 12	> 400	> 400
Transferrin (mg/dl)	360	> 360	>> 360	normal– ↓	normal– ↓
Iron absorption	↑	↑	↑	↑	↓
Erythrocytes	normal	normal	microcytic	normal	normal
Sideroblasts (%)	40–60	< 10	< 10	40-60	40-60

Prelatent Iron Deficiency

Prelatent iron deficiency, which is equivalent to storage iron deficiency, is characterized by a negative iron balance. The body's reaction is to increase the intestinal absorption of iron. Histochemically, the iron content of bone marrow and of liver tissue decreases. The concentration of the iron transport protein transferrin in the blood increases as a measure of the increased intestinal absorption.

The consumption of storage iron is most easily detected by quantitative determination of the ferritin concentration, which typically falls to less than 20 ng/ml. The ferritin that can be detected in the circulating blood is directly related to the iron stores, and can thus be used as an indicator. The determination of ferritin has almost entirely replaced the determination of iron in bone marrow for the assessment of stocks of reserve iron [111].

Latent Iron Deficiency

With increasing consumption of reserve iron, or when the iron stores are completely empty, the replenishment of iron for erythropoiesis becomes negative. The total loss of storage iron is indicated by a decrease in the ferritin concentration to less than 12 ng/ml. An indication of the inadequate supply of iron for erythropoiesis is a decrease in the transferrin saturation to less than 15%. As a morphological criterion, the number of sideroblasts in the marrow falls to less than 10%. There are no noticeable changes in the red blood count at this stage of latent iron deficiency.

Manifest Iron Deficiency: Iron Deficiency Anemia

In addition to the decrease of the ferritin concentration to less than 12 ng/ml, the laboratory results in this stage are characterized by a fall in the hemoglobin concentration to less than 12 g/dl. A morphological effect of manifest iron deficiency is that the erythrocytes become increasingly hypochromic and microcytic. The mean cell volume (MCV) decreases to less than 85 fl, the mean cellular hemoglobin (MCH) is less than 27 pg and the mean cellular hemoglobin concentration (MCHC) may fall to less than 31 g/dl. The erythrocytes in the peripheral blood count are smaller than normal, and pale in the center. The altered erythrocytes are known as anulocytes. The morphological change in the blood count does not appear immediately, but only after the normochromic erythrocyte population has been replaced by the hypochromic microcytic erythrocytes in the course of the natural process of renewal. Iron deficiency is by no means ruled out by normochromic normocytic anemia. Pronounced hypochromia and microcythemia indicate that the iron deficiency has already been in existence for at least several months (Table 12). A hypochromic microcytic anemia is not necessarily an iron deficiency anemia. However, a hypochromic microcytic anemia accompanied by a ferritin value of less than 12 ng/ml can always be identified as an iron deficiency anemia, and there is then, for the present, no need for further tests.

Differential Diagnosis of Iron Deficiency

It is extremely important in differential diagnosis to distinguish between the common iron deficiency anemias and other hypochromic anemias, since this has considerable implications for therapy. Only iron deficiency anemia responds to iron replacement. For patients suffering from other hypochromic anemias, the unnecessary administration of iron would lead to a risk of iron overload.

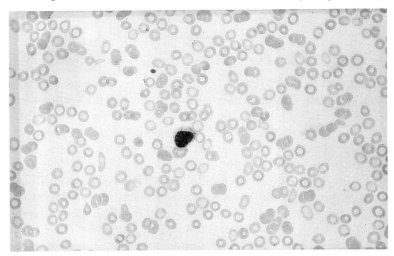

Fig. 21. Anulocytes

Differential diagnostic possibilities to consider for hypochromic anemia are chronic anemias due to infections or tumors, sideroblastic anemia, and thalassemia. The most important distinguishing feature is the quantity of reserve iron. These forms of anemia can be identified on the basis of the ferritin concentration, since they all differ from true iron deficiency anemia in that the storage iron concentrations are normal or increased (Fig. 22).

It is possible for an infection-related or tumor-related anemia or a thalassemia to be combined with iron deficiency anemia. In all such cases, the ferritin determination shows that the iron stores are low, and that iron therapy is justified.

Clinical Pictures of Iron Deficiency

Iron deficiency occurs as a sign of increased physiological iron requirements during growth [116], as a result of menstruation, in pregnancy, and during breast-feeding. The main cause of pathological iron deficiency, on the other hand, is loss of blood, usually from the gastrointestinal tract, though also from the urogenital tract in the case of women, and less commonly in both

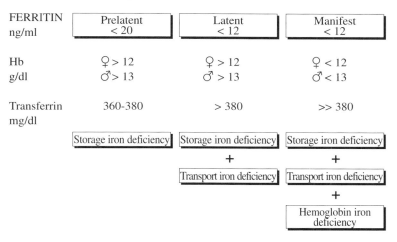

FERRITIN ng/ml	Prelatent < 20	Latent < 12	Manifest < 12
Hb g/dl	♀ > 12 ♂ > 13	♀ > 12 ♂ > 13	♀ < 12 ♂ < 13
Transferrin mg/dl	360-380	> 380	>> 380
	Storage iron deficiency	Storage iron deficiency **+** Transport iron deficiency	Storage iron deficiency **+** Transport iron deficiency **+** Hemoglobin iron deficiency

Fig. 22. Iron deficiency

sexes as a result of renal and bladder hemorrhages. Iron deficiency can also be caused by malabsorption of iron, in which case it is important to check for any medication that interferes with the absorption of iron. The clinical pictures of latent or manifest iron deficiency following blood loss are relatively easy to detect by a detailed patient history or by appropriate diagnostic measures. Checks for occult blood in the stools are particularly important in the case of gastrointestinal losses.

Iatrogenic iron deficiency may be caused by excessive laboratory tests or by drugs, such as non-steroidal antirheumatic drugs or antacids. Asymptomatic gastrointestinal losses due to corticosteroids also fall under this heading.

Frequent blood donations (e.g., 2 to 4 times within a year) empty the iron stores. Further donations then lead to a reduced -but constant- ferritin concentration. Males donating 4 or more times per year and females donating 2 or more per year should have at least one ferritin determination per year, to allow for detection and treatment of any prelatent or latent iron deficiency .

Table 13. Causes of iron deficiency

1. Physiological increase in requirements	• Tumors of the urinary tract
• Growth phase	Calculi
• Menstruation	• Iatrogenic
• Pregnancy	Laboratory testing (excessive)
• Breast-feeding	Drugs
	Blood donors
2. Blood loss	3. Malabsorption
• Gastrointestinal	• Sprue
Varices	• Gastric resections
Ulcers	• Chronic atrophic gastritis
Tumors	• Drugs
Inflammations	
Malformation (blood vessels)	4. Inadequate supply
• Urogenital	• Unbalanced diet
Hypermenorrhea	• Old age
Birth	• New vegetarians

Disturbances of iron absorption are known to occur after gastric resections (often associated with vitamin B_{12} deficiency) and in chronic atrophic gastritis. Malabsorption may also be induced iatrogenically by long-term tetracycline therapy, such as is often used for the treatment of acne. Idiopathic sprue generally also leads to iron malabsorption and hence to anemia.

Special consideration must also be given to certain population groups in which iron deficiency is common; these include infants and adolescents, the elderly, competitive athletes, and individuals having an unbalanced diet.

Behavioral disturbances in children can often be traced to latent or manifest iron deficiency. Intellectual and especially cognitive development in childhood is also adversely affected by iron deficiency. The observed symptoms can be eliminated by oral administration of iron. There is some debate as to whether brain development is permanently damaged by iron deficiency in early childhood. Iron deficiency in adolescence, especially in girls, is aggravated by poor eating habits. The supply of iron often corresponds to only 50% of the recommended amount, and this, coupled with puberty, leads to iron deficiency [116].

Latent iron deficiency is found in more than 50% of all pregnant women. The physiological course of pregnancy explains why latent iron deficiency appears mainly in the final three months. The ferritin concentration is a reliable parameter for the detection of iron depletion and deficiency in this situation. The daily iron requirement increases to 5-6 mg during the last three months of pregnancy, and this amount cannot be absorbed even from the best possible diet. Oral iron replacement is therefore necessary (Fig. 23).

Iron deficiency in the elderly, particularly those who live alone or in an institution, appears to be caused mainly by diet [120].

Special note should given to iron deficiency in athletes of both sexes who take part in endurance sports. Iron deficiency in runners is mainly due to gastro-intestinal looses after long-distance running. Latent iron deficiency has also been found in long-distance swimmers. In endurance sports apparently a hemolytic influence is an additional factor [116].

Extremely unbalanced diets have recently attracted considerable numbers of adherents. Iron deficiency anemia develops here mainly if the diet has an extremely high content of indigestible roughage [13].

Iron Overload – Elevated Ferritin Concentrations

The human body is incapable of actively excreting excess iron. An over-abundant supply of iron leads to increased concentrations of the iron storage proteins ferritin and hemosiderin. If the

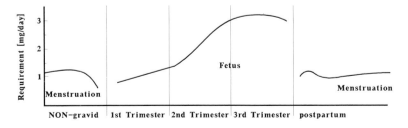

Fig. 23. Iron requirement during pregnancy

storage capacity is exceeded, deposition takes place in the parenchymatous organs. The resulting cell damage leads to cell death and to functional impairment of the organ in question.

It has been suggested that this damage is due to toxic effects of free iron ions on the enzyme metabolism and to lysosome damage.

Iron overload, unlike iron deficiency, is rare. However, it is often overlooked or misinterpreted, and can progress to a life-threatening stage as a result. An elevated ferritin level should always suggest an iron overload, and the possibility of a true iron overload should be explored by differential diagnosis. On the other hand, disturbances of iron distribution must also be considered as a possibility (Fig. 24).

Representative Ferritin Increase

Iron storage diseases can be divided into a primary HLA-associated form, known as idiopathic hemochromatosis, and various secondary forms, or acquired hemochromatoses. The secondary forms are also known as hemosideroses.

Primary Hemochromatosis

In primary hereditary HLA-associated hemochromatosis [38], an autosomal recessive disturbance of iron metabolism is apparent which can lead to severe parenchymal iron overload. The

Table 14. Causes of iron overload

---

1. Primary (hereditary) hemochromatosis

2. Secondary (acquired) hemochromatosis
   - Ineffective erythropoiesis
     Thalassemia major
     Sideroblastic anemias
     Aplastic anemias
   - Transfusions

3. Dietary
   - Extreme ingestion of iron
     African dietary ironoverload
     Chronic alcoholism

IRON OVERLOAD

Representative	Non-representative
Ferritin > 400 ng/ml	Ferritin > 400 ng/ml
Transferrin Saturation >50%	Transferrin Saturation ↓
	Transferrin ↓
Confirmation of Diagnosis	Confirmation of Diagnosis

by:

Clinical Examination
Case History
PCR
Biopsy
Intestinal iron absorbtion
HLA Typing

by:

Clinical Examination
Case History

| Hemochromatoses | Disturbance of Distribution Release Increased Synthesis? |

↓ = reduced

Fig. 24. Differential diagnosis of conditions with elevated ferritin.

genetic defect is situated in a gene mutation on the short arm of chromosome 6 (HFE gene) and causes increased iron absorption in the small intestine and increased storage in the affected organs, namely the parenchymal cells of the liver, the heart, the pancreas, and the adrenal glands with the appropriate accompanying clinical complications such as diabetes, cirrhosis of the liver, arthropathy, cardiomyopathy and impotence.

The transport protein for iron, DTC 1, is mainly localized in the duodenum within the enterocytic membrane and increases in concentration during alimentary iron deficiency. DTC 1 is also expressed in the kidneys, liver, brain and heart.

The HFE genetic product is localized in the gastrointestinal tract and in the mutated form it is not capable of migrating out of the cell [38].

The prevalence of the disease is between 4 and 14% in Europe with a significant divide between North and South.

Men are affected approximately 10 times more often than women by primary hemochromatosis which becomes clinically manifest between the ages of 35 and 55 and causes liver function disorders, diabetes mellitus, dark pigmentation of the skin, cardiomyopathy and resulting arrhythmia. Furthermore, complaints of the joints and symptoms due to secondary hypogonadism as well as adrenal gland insufficiency have been observed. In about 15% of those affected by the illness, liver cell carcinoma arises which represents a 300-fold risk.

In primary hemochromatosis, the plasma ferritin level rises at a relatively late stage. Initially parenchymal cells of the liver, heart and pancreas as well as other organs are overloaded with iron and only thereafter is the reticuloendothelial system saturated. Ferritin values above 400 ng/ml and a transferrin saturation of more than 50% signify existing iron overload. In the manifest stage of primary hemochromatosis, ferritin concentrations in serum are usually over 700 ng/ml. Transferrin is almost completely saturated.

A biopsy was necessary in the past to conclusively diagnose primary hyperchromatosis (liver biopsy being the most appropriate) but a major advance has been made recently by the advent of identifying specific genetic changes for diagnosing the disease. The genetic defect can be identified using a molecular biological test.

Hemochromatosis can be identified in 80% of the cases using the simple and relatively economically feasible PCR and DNA sequencing technologies before the manifestation of clinical symptoms. This opens up the possibility of timely treatment such that late-stage complications like cirrhosis of the liver and cancer of the liver can be prevented.

As was the case in the past, the therapy of choice is still phlebotomy. The aim of the therapy is to deplete iron stores as much as possible. The determination of the body iron status should be performed frequently at short intervals and in hereditary hemochromatosis the determination of plasma ferritin has proven to be of worth. The progression of the clinical parameter determines the necessity of continuing phlebotomy therapy. Phlebotomy at weekly, monthly or quarterly intervals may be necessary, however the therapy should never completely cease. As described above, the aim of phlebotomy is to prevent a negative progression of the disease. Early identification of patients at risk which has become possible by virtue of the molecular biological detection of genetic defects can probably drastically reduce the incidence of hepatocellular carcinomas.

Secondary Hemochromatosis

Hematopoietic disorders with concomitant ineffective or hypoplastic erythropoiesis such as thalassemia major, sideroblastic anemia or aplastic anemia are considered to be secondary or acquired hemochromatoses.

Acquired hemochromatoses can also develop from alimentary iron overload, parenteral administration of iron and transfusions or other chronic diseases with ineffective erythrocytopoiesis.

Alcoholics with chronic liver disease in whom iron deposits have been detected after liver biopsies but whose total body iron levels are within the non-pathological range present a particular diagnostic challenge. Such patients probably suffer from an alcohol-induced liver disease (toxic nutritive cirrhosis) and seem to acquire iron deposits as a result of cell necroses and iron uptake from such necrotic cells.

However, a second group of alcoholics has been identified who have extremely high deposits of iron in their bodies and massive iron deposits in the cirrhotic liver. Such patients may suffer from congenital primary hemochromatosis with concomitant toxic nutritive liver disease.

The molecular biological detection of causative primary hemochromatosis makes differential diagnosis more straight forward.

Patients suffering from renal insufficiency on dialysis were first treated with erythropoietin in 1988 and for this group of patients iron overloading caused by transfusions should belong firmly to the past.

In contrast to primary hemochromatosis in the secondary form the cells of the reticuloendothelial system are initially overloaded with iron. Organ damage occurs at a relatively late stage. They arise because of a redistribution of iron from the cells of the reticuloendothelial system into parenchymal cells of individual organs. The duration of chronic iron overloading in secondary iron storage disorders is therefore a critical factor.

Disturbances of Iron Distribution

Non-Representative Raised Plasma Ferritin Concentrations

While the plasma ferritin concentration correlates with the body's total iron reserves in patients with primary and secondary hemochromatoses, there are other conditions in which this correlation does not apply. Raised plasma ferritin concentrations are also found in patients with infection or toxin-induced damage to liver cells resulting from ferritin release in liver cell necroses, in patients with latent and manifest inflammations or infections, and in patients with rheumatoid arthritis. Raised plasma ferritin concentrations are also observed in patients suffering from physical and psychological stress, e.g. following serious trauma. In critically ill patients, plasma ferritin concentrations increase with increasing deterioration of the patient's clinical status, probably as a result of increased release from the macrophage system [11].

The plasma ferritin concentration is not indicative of the body's total iron reserves shortly after oral or parenteral iron therapy, or in patients with malignant tumors. As a basic rule, it can be assumed that a raised red blood cell sedimentation rate and/or pathological values for C-reactive protein are likely to be accompanied by raised plasma ferritin concentrations.

Anemia of Chronic Disorders (ACD)

Disturbances of iron distribution and resultant anemia are observed in patients with chronic infections and chronic autoimmune diseases. This form of anemia – along with iron deficiency anemia – is the most common. In addition to chronic inflammatory and neoplastic processes, it is observed primarily in patients with extensive tissue trauma.

The characteristics of this anemia that can be determined using laboratory-based methods are low serum iron concentrations combined with low transferrin saturation. The iron storage protein ferritin is available in sufficient or elevated quantities. The morphology of the anemia is normocytic or microcytic.

Transferrin concentrations and reticulocyte count are usually normal or slightly reduced, while the concentration of the transferrin receptor is slightly elevated.

The pathogenesis of ACD is affected by very diverse factors, the most important of which are cytokines produced by CD4+T-helper cells [138]. Additionally, disturbances of iron distribution are affected by short-lived radicals (H_2O_2, NO), acute-phase proteins, and hormones, as well as by factors that induce ACD (bacteria, toxins, TNF-α).

While a subpopulation of cd4+T helper cells (TH1) releases pro-inflammatory cytokines, which have a direct effect on iron metabolism, the TH2 population is mainly responsible for the antibody response.

The cytokines produced by TH1 subsets, such as interleukin-1 and TNF-α, induce ferritin synthesis in macrophages and hepatocytes by means of a transcription mechanism, while interferon gamma withholds iron from the macrophages. Contrary to the TH1 subpopulation, the TH2 cells that stimulate the antibody response produce cytokines that promote iron uptake and storage in activated macrophages.

Short-lived radicals (H_2O_2, NO) and iron deficiency promote cellular iron uptake and inhibit the consumption and storage of iron and stimulation of iron responsive elements (IRE).

Conversely, inhibited production of radicals leads to inhibited iron uptake, iron consumption, and iron storage.

Cytokines can overwhelm the effect of these radicals on iron metabolism, because there is a form of NO synthesis (NOS type II) induced by cytokines, the production of which in the nucleus can overwhelm cytoplasmic activity.

In macrophages themselves, the equilibrium between iron homeostasis and NO formation is in most cases controlled by means of autoregulatory mechanisms – a direct intervention into the immune system.

NO inhibits biosynthesis by inhibiting the ceruloplasmin/haptoglobin system, and also directly inhibits the proliferation of precursor cells of erythropoiesis.

Iron and Cellular Immunity

Iron intervenes in cellular immunity at many levels [141]. On the one hand, it affects the proliferation and differentiation of various lymphocyte subsets. On the other, it affects the immunopotential of macrophages [14, 25] by blocking the INF-γ-transmitted immune response in macrophages [139].

Iron-overloaded macrophages react more poorly to INF-γ, produce more TNF-α, and form more NO. This weakens the resistance to viruses and other intracellular pathogens. The withdrawal of metabolically active iron and its deposit as storage iron (which is typical in ACD) strengthens the organism's immune response to INF-γ stimulation [1, 5, 71, 92].

The regulatory antagonist of this stimulation mechanism lies in the reduction of the TH1-mediated immune reaction by IL-4 and IL-13. This is accomplished when these interleukins raise the intracellular concentration of iron by stimulating transferrin receptor expression. This is one of the basic mechanisms of the anti-inflammatory and macrophage-inhibiting effect.

Since iron is an important factor in the growth of tissue and microorganisms, iron deficiency limits DNA synthesis. Additionally, reduced hemoglobin synthesis and erythropoiesis is associated with a reduction in oxygen transport capacity, which has a negative effect on the supply of oxygen to rapidly growing tissues and microorganisms.

Iron, Acute-Phase Proteins, and Hormones

The effect of cytokines (IL-1, IL-6) on ferritin-MRNA is interpreted as a part of the acute-phase reaction. By means of iron storage in the hepatocyte toxic reactions by radicals are inhibited.

It has been demonstrated that the acute-phase proteins alpha$_1$-antitrypsin and alpha$_2$-macroglobulin can inhibit transferrin receptor-controlled iron uptake in erythroblasts and hepatocytes, but not in monocytes [44, 139].

The effect of hormones on iron metabolism is partially understood for thyroid hormones. There are indications that they affect ferritin synthesis in liver cells. The extent to which they affect disturbances of iron metabolism in ACD is unknown, however [78, 79].

Other factors in the development of ACD are bacterial toxins and various cytokines (e.g., TNF-α), which shorten the survival time of erythrocytes and accelerate their culling by the spleen.

Additionally, cytokines negatively influence the proliferation and differentiation of erythrocytic precursors by decreasing erythropoietin sensitivity which, in turn, lowers erythropoietin production [45, 90].

Various pathogens can also suppress erythropoiesis directly, as is the case in HIV and malaria plasmodia [12, 148].

Anemias of Rheumatoid Arthritis (RA)

Due to a chronic inflammatory process, rheumatoid arthritis leads to the gradual, progressive destruction of joint cartilage

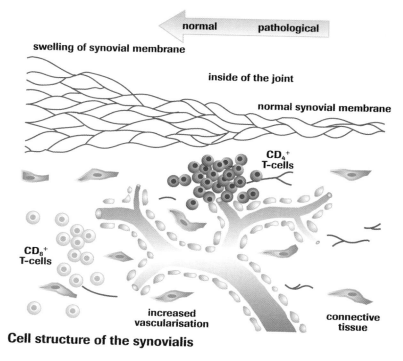

Fig. 25. Cell structure of the synovialis

and bone. The disease is not limited to joints, however. It is also frequently manifested in other organs such as the heart, eyes, and kidneys.

In every case, the joints become inflamed. This inflammation is accompanied by a strong, painful swelling of the synovial membrane. Connective tissue then proliferates in the cartilage, which eventually destroys the joint cartilage and the exposed bone. In cases of pronounced activity, the patient also suffers from anemia and thrombocytosis.

Neutrophils accumulate in the synovial fluid, while macrophages and T-lymphocytes in particular accumulate in the

Table 15. Laboratory diagnosis of rheumatic diseases

	CRP	RF	ASL, ADNASE	ANA
Rheumatoid arthritis	++	++	−	+
Rheumatic fever	+	(+)	++	(+)
Collagen disease, e.g. SLE	(+)	(+)	−	+++

RF	= Rheumatoid factor
CRP	= C-reactive protein
ASL	= Antistreptolysin titer
ADNASE	= Streptodornase
ANA	= Antinuclear antibody
SLE	= Systemic Lupus Erythematodes

synovial membrane. Cell infiltration and the regeneration of blood vessels cause the synovial membrane to thicken (formation of pannus). During this process, large quantities of macrophages are located in the border of the synovial membrane and in the cartilage contact zone. The macrophages and fibroblasts are induced via proinflammatory cytokines (e.g., TNF-α, IL-1) to release collagenase and stromelysin 1, two matrix metalloproteinases that play a significant role in the destruction of cartilage. Osteoclasts are stimulated.

Excess quantities of released tumor necrosis factor alpha (TNF-α) play a central role in the development of inflammation and joint destruction in the induction of rheumatoid arthritis. Two new principles of action are now available to neutralize raised levels of TNF-α: TNF-α antibodies such as Infliximab (Remicade®), and soluble TNF receptors such as Etanercept (Enbrel®) [118].

The use of anti-inflammatory substances such as nonsteroidal anti-rheumatics, glucocorticoids, antimetabolites (methotrexate), and immunosuppressants has been established for years to treat chronic polyarthritis. Inhibition of tumor necrosis factor alpha (TNF-α) is a new therapeutic concept. TNF-α occurs at the beginning of a cascade of cytokines that eventually lead to inflammation and tissue destruction.

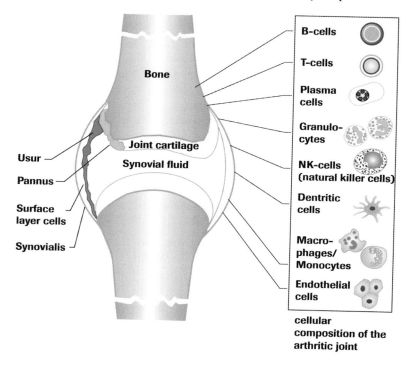

Fig. 26. Cells in the arthritic joint
(According to Burmester G (1998) Taschenatlas der Immunologie: Grundlagen Labor, Klinik. Thieme, Stuttgart, New York)

Iron metabolism in monocytes/macrophages plays an especially significant role in chronic disease. The organism uses iron
metabolism in the inflammatory and anti-neoplastic defense system. It draws iron from microorganisms and neoplastic cells and
stores it in reticuloendothelial systems. This is characterized by
the development of normochromic, normocytic anemia (ACD,
anemias of chronic disease). This type of anemia is caused by all
types of inflammation (rheumatoid arthritis, malignant growths,
or trauma). Due to various cytokines, erythropoiesis is compromised primarily at the CFU-E level in this process.

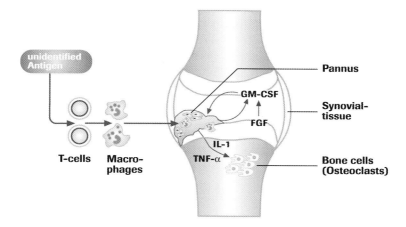

Fig. 27. Induction of rheumatoid arthritis
(According to Burmester G (1998) Taschenatlas der Immuno-
logie: Grundlagen Labor, Klinik. Thieme, Stuttgart, New York)
FGF = Fibroblast growth factor
GM-CSF = Granulocyte macrophage/monocyte
colony-stimulating factor

TNF-α (tumor necrosis factor) induces stroma cells to form
inhibitory IFN-β (interferon), thereby indirectly suppressing the
formation of CFU-E.

IL-1 (interleukin) induces the IFN-γ synthesis of T-cells.
IFN-γ also suppresses CFU-E.

Monocytes/macrophages play an important role in erythropoiesis in bone marrow [141].

The progenitor cells of the red line proliferate and differentiate only under optimal local conditions [141].

The blood islands in bone marrow consist of a centrally located macrophage surrounded by small cells of the erythroid and
myeloid line. The surrounding cells also comprise endothelial
cells, fat cells, reticuloepithelial cells, and fibroblasts.

Erythropoietin (EPO) is the most important and specific erythropoiesis-stimulating factor. It acts on early progenitor cells up

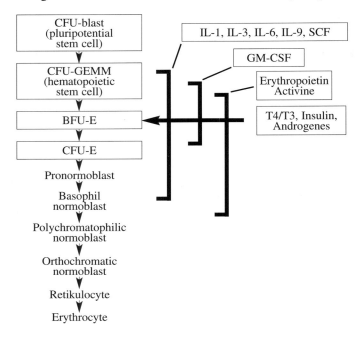

Fig. 28. Differentiation of the hematopoetic system and regulation of the erythropoiesis by growth factors
CFU = Colonie forming unit, **BFU** = Burst forming unit,
E = Erythrocytic, **G** = Granulocytic, **M** = Macrophagocytic,
M = Megaloblastic **IL** = Interleukin, **SCF** = Stem cell factor,
GM-CSF = Granulocyte-macrophage colony-stimulating factor
] = Effektivness of growth factors

to the maturation levels after the erythroblast. Without EPO, erythroid differentiation does not progress past the level of burst forming units (BFU-E).

High concentrations of intracellular iron dramatically reduce the effect of IFN-γ on human monocytic cells. Iron regulates the cytokine effects in this process.

Macrophages with high concentrations of intracellular iron loose the ability to phagocyt. After stimulation with IFN-γ and lipopolysaccharides (LPS), cultivated macrophages produce increasing quantities of nitrogen oxide (NO), which is then converted to reactive nitrogen intermediates (RNI) such as nitrite and nitrate.

Since the introduction of tumor necrosis factor receptor-blocking substances (e.g., Infliximab) and fusion proteins for TNF-α (e.g., Etanacept), it has been possible to rapidly decrease RA activity. The indication for treatment with these substances is extremely limited (de novo-lymphomas resulting from therapy are discussed) [118].

Improved clinical symptoms accompany a significant improvement in the anemia.

Other cytokines, such as IFN-α, IL-6, and TGF-β, which play an important role in autoimmune-inflammatory events, are also capable of effectively inhibiting erythropoiesis in vivo and are probably involved in the formation of ACD.

Erythropoietin (EPO) is the central growth factor for the regulation of erythropoiesis and represents a new starting point for the treatment of ACD. With this form of anemia, EPO exhibits a positive correlation with the extent of the anemia, i.e., it increases as hemoglobin concentration decreases. In patients with rheumatoid arthritis, however, who can be considered a model population for ACD, the EPO level remains clearly below that of patients without RA but with the same intensity of anemia of a different origin [141].

Although the insufficient increase in EPO in patients with RA contributes to reduced erythropoiesis in ACD, the primary cause cannot be considered to be the relative EPO deficiency alone, because the concentrations measured in anemic RA patients are still higher than those measured in non-anemic, healthy individuals. Rather, the inability of the bone marrow to adequately respond to EPO in the presence of an inflammatory systemic disease must be considered the cause of the ACD. No evidence for decreased bioactivity of EPO exists to date. In vitro studies suggest, however, that mediators released during inflammatory processes are at least partially capable of inhibiting the EPO effect [138].

This discussion of ACD can be summed up by saying that the interaction between a direct effect on iron metabolism and alteration of cellular immunity leads clinically to the development of a functional iron deficiency which is important with regard to the appropriate therapy. The fact that erythropoietin production cannot be stimulated in patients with collagen disease [72] is an additional factor which influences the therapy.

Anemias in Malignant Neoplasia (Erythropoietin as Tumor Marker)

Autonomous erythropoietin production has also been observed in renal-cell carcinoma and as a paraneoplastic phenomenon. However, these phenomena are also seen in Wilms' tumors, hepatocellular cancer and cerebellar angioblastomas [87]. In a few cases a drop in the erythropoietin level has been observed after surgical procedures, and a rise when the tumor developed metastases or there was a local recurrence. The measurement of erythropoietin levels in erythropoietin-producing tumors is limited to monitoring and checking the outcome of treatment [88].

Disturbances of Iron Utilization

In spite of all the studies carried out since it has been possible to determine the transferrin receptor in the blood and the erythron transferrin uptake, the mechanism of disturbance of iron utilization in uremic and dialysis patients has remained largely unexplained.

One thing is certain and that is that in uremic patients, transferrin receptor determination in the plasma is approximately 35% below the mean for healthy control subjects. This mean value correlates well with the erythron transferrin uptake, provided that there are adequate iron reserves. In principle, patients with chronic renal failure behave like normal healthy control subjects, but at an approximately 40% lower level [36, 59].

Erythropoietin

Erythropoietin is a glycoprotein with a molecular weight of 34,000 daltons and consists of 165 amino acids. Its protein component comprises two disulfide bonds which are among other things responsible for the biological activity. The tertiary structure of erythropoietin is unknown.

Oxygen shortage stimulates erythropoietin production. Goldberg et al. [43] have postulated that a hemoprotein serves as renal oxygen sensor for this mechanism. Fischer et al. discuss the possibility of a reduction in oxygen tension. This leads to the release of adenosine which, as messenger substance, activates adenylate cyclase via a cascade which leads to increased erythropoietin production and erythropoietin secretion. Also shunts in the renal cortex influence erythropoietin production [104]. The site of erythropoietin production in the kidney is also unknown: all working groups agree that erythropoietin is produced in the renal cortex and not the glomerular system. More recent studies have shown that a subpopulation of macrophages produces erythropoietin outside the kidney. A difference between the erythropoietin production of the kidney and that of the macrophages could be due to differences in oxygen sensitivity.

The clinical finding that plasma erythropoietin is lower in uremic patients than in non-uremic patients with a comparable degree of anemia suggests that the kidney is the main producer of erythropoietin. Studies of iron kinetics have revealed a disturbance in iron incorporation. It is therefore legitimate to talk of ineffective erythropoiesis.

In this connection the question arises of whether the determination of *erythropoietin* is useful in *clinical diagnostics*. The determination of serum erythropoietin can in principle be used in the differential diagnosis of erythrocytosis, to check for paraneoplastic erythropoietin production, in the differential diagnosis of anemia and finally also for diagnosis in patients who apparently have non-renal anemia and have adequate iron depots. The determination of erythropoietin can thus be used in the differential diagnosis of erythrocytosis of uncertain etiology and anemia. In particular, diagnosis to differentiate between polycythemia vera, where suppression of erythropoietin is expected, and secondary erythrocytosis (lung diseases, cardiac decompensation) where increased erythropoietin production is expected, is useful. But there is evidence that in certain patients determination is without consequence. Extremely high erythropoietin levels have been observed in aplastic anemia and other forms of medullary hyperplasia [34].

Uremic Anemia

Uremic anemia is an important special form of normochromic normocytic anemia. It correlates roughly with the course of azotemia. By contrast, the cause of the kidney failure clearly plays a more secondary role, although patients with polycystic kidney disease for a long time have a normal blood count or less pronounced anemia than patients with kidney disease of a different origin. The striking fact is that uremic anemia is amazingly well tolerated by patients, and hemoglobin levels as low as 5 g/dl are tolerated with relatively few symptoms. Most patients' reticulocyte count is low and the survival time of the red blood cells is only moderately reduced. The anemia is thus the result of a massive disturbance of erythrocyte production in the bone marrow.

The introduction of the transferrin receptor determination has not shed light on the pathogenesis of uremic anemias. As has already been mentioned elsewhere, insofar as their functions in adequate ferritin depots is concerned, the transferrin receptors in the plasma behave as they do in healthy subjects, but at a considerably lower level [36, 59].

This is not surprising if we bear in mind that the main production centers of the transferrin receptor are the immature cells of erythropoiesis, which are reduced in mass in chronic renal failure. Therefore it would appear that serum transferrin receptor production in renal anemias is also dependent on erythropoietin.

Although uremic anemia is obviously multifactorial in origin and can be partially improved by appropriate hemodialysis therapy, the role played by the extracorporeal hemolytic component must not be underestimated. Some patients have developed a defect in the hexose monophosphatase shunt; in addition, influences in hemodialysis such as mechanical intravascular hemolysis or pump trauma play an increasing role.

If there are adequate ferritin depots, uremic anemia can be slightly improved by hemodialysis. In the past it has generally been fully corrected in a very short time by a successful kidney transplant. The erythrocytosis occasionally observed following transplantation is considered to be a sign of an incipient rejection reaction [16].

The treatment of renal anemia was revolutionized by the development and introduction of recombinant human erythropoietin [46]. If sufficient depot iron is available, which clinical experience shows as requiring ferritin levels of at least 100 ng/ml, uremic anemia can be corrected. As mentioned before, transferrin saturation should be at least 30% as indication of functional available iron. The adjustment of the erythropoietin dose to the individual needs of the patient and subcutaneous administration [89], with the aim of achieving a hemoglobin level of between 10 and 11 g/dl, prevents the unpleasant side effects observed initially, such as hypertension and dialysis shunt thrombosis.

Since the folic acid deficiency in dialysis patients can contribute to the development of anemia, care should be taken to maintain sufficiently high depot iron reserves and to avoid a folic acid deficit. Changed iron kinetics or aluminum accumulations may delay or inhibit the action of erythropoietin.

Non-iron-induced Disturbances of Erythropoiesis

Deficiencies in vitamin B_{12}, folic acid and erythropoietin have been found to be crucial factors in non-iron-deficiency-induced forms of anemia.

An initial diagnosis can be made with a high degree of accuracy by recording the patient's history or from knowledge of the primary disease. Given the known interaction between vitamin B_{12} and folic acid, the determination of these two cofactors by immunoassay should now be standard clinical practice.

Deficiency in folic acid or vitamin B_{12} is the main feature of diseases accompanied by macrocytic anemia.

Sternal puncture or bone biopsies also offer clear histological and morphological pictures.

In the differential diagnosis of macrocytic anemia, an elevated level of LDH with simultaneous reticulocytosis and hyperbilirubinemia (both to be interpreted as hyperregeneratory anemia) directs attention to a vitamin B_{12} deficit. Macrocytic anemia without these components makes a genuine folic acid deficiency likely (pregnancy, alcohol).

Normocytic forms of anemia draw attention to the hemolytic component of erythrocyte destruction, with haptoglobin playing the crucial role as the key to diagnosis. Erythrocyte morphology provides a means to exclude mechanical hemolysis or to look for hemoglobinopathy (Hb electrophoresis) or an enzyme defect.

Proof of impaired renal function makes it likely that the most important deficiency of a cofactor in Hb synthesis is present, a deficiency of erythropoietin.

The determination of erythropoietin which can now be performed by immunoassay at least forms a good base for a prognosis of the outcome of treatment. Before giving any treatment with erythropoietin, it is important to determine the iron depots, since otherwise action by the parenterally administered erythropoietin, which is genetically engineered today, is impossible.

Table 16. Deficiencies in the cofactors of erythropoiesis

Microcytic anemia	Macrocytic anemia	Normocytic anemia
Iron metabolism disturbances	Folic acid deficiency	Renal anemia
ACD		
Hemoglobinopathies	B_{12} deficiency	Hemolytic anemia
	Drug-induced	
	Metabolic disease	Hemoglobinopathies
	Uncertain origin	Bone marrow diseases
		Toxic bone marrow damage

In summary it can be said that, given adequate iron depots, normocytic forms of anemia with normal or reduced reticulocyte counts (= disturbance of erythrocyte production) justify looking for erythropoietin deficiency.

Macrocytic Anemia

A non-representative ferritin increase may indicate disturbances in the proliferation and maturation of bone marrow cells induced by vitamin deficiency.

These macrocytic forms of anemia are caused by disturbed DNA synthesis. As non-iron-induced disturbances of erythropoiesis, they influence not only the proliferation of cells of erythropoiesis, but above all that of the gastrointestinal epithelial cells. Since considerable numbers of macrocytic cells are destroyed while still in the bone marrow, they are also included under the heading ineffective erythropoiesis.

Most macrocytic forms of anemia are due to a deficiency in either vitamin B_{12} or folic acid, or both. The most common causes of folic acid and vitamin B_{12} deficiency are listed in Tables 17 and 18.

Table 17. Drug-induced forms of macrocytic anemia

1. Drugs which act via folic acid
   - Malabsorption
   alcohol, phenytoin, barbiturates
   - Metabolism
   alcohol, methotrexate, pyrimethamine, triamterene, pentamidine
2. Drugs which act via vitamin B_{12}
   - PAS, colchicine, neomycin
3. Inhibitors of DNA metabolism
   - Purine antagonists (azathioprine, 6-mercaptopurine)
   - Pyrimidine antagonists (5-fluorouracil, cytosine arabinoside)
   - Others
   (procarbazine, acyclovir, zidovudine, hydroxyurea)

Table 18. Symptomatic forms of macrocytic anemia

1. Metabolic diseases
   - Aciduria (orotic acid)
2. Uncertain origin
   - Di-Guglielmo syndrome
   - Congenital dyserythropoietic anemia
   - Refractory megaloblastic anemia

Drug-induced macrocytic anemia is now common (Table 17). Drugs which disturb DNA synthesis are now part of the standard therapeutic armamentarium of chemotherapy. There are also rare metabolic disturbances which cause macrocytic anemia, plus megaloblastic anemia with as yet unknown causes, such as the congenital dyserythropoietic anemias or anemias as part of the Di-Guglielmo syndrome (Table 18).

Acute severe macrocytic anemia is a rarity; it can be observed in intensive care patients who require multiple transfusions, hemodialysis or total parenteral nutrition.

This form of acute macrocytic anemia may be limited mainly to patients who already had borderline folic acid depots before they fell ill.

Folic Acid Deficiency

Patients with a folic acid deficit are usually in a poor nutritional state, and often have a range of gastrointestinal symptoms such as diarrhea, cheilosis and glossitis. In contrast to advanced vitamin B_{12} deficiency no neurological deficits are found.

Folic acid deficiency can be attributed to three main causes: inadequate intake, increased requirement, and malabsorption.

Special attention must be devoted to various groups in the population who commonly have inadequate folic acid intake: chronic alcoholics, the elderly, and adolescents.

In chronic alcoholics, the alcohol which is the main source of energy (beer and wine) contains practically no folic acid or only small quantities. Alcohol also leads to disturbances in the processing of absorbed folic acid [126].

Table 19. Causes of Folic Acid Deficiency

1. Inadequate intake
   - Alcoholism
   - Unbalanced diet
2. Increased requirement
   - Pregnancy
   - Adolescence
   - Malignancy
   - Increased cell turnover
     (hemolysis, chronic exfoliative skin diseases)
   - Hemodialysis patients?
3. Malabsorption
   - Sprue
   - Drugs (barbiturates, phenytoin)
4. Disturbed folic acid metabolism
   - Inhibition of dihydrofolic acid reductase
     (methotrexate, pyrimethamin, triamterene)
   - Congenital enzyme defects

The folic acid deficit in the elderly seems to be caused mainly by an extremely unbalanced diet ("coffee and a sandwich").

Unbalanced diets have a considerable attraction for adolescents. Those who consume fast food are particularly at risk.

An increased folic acid requirement is present during the growth phase in childhood and adolescence, as well as during pregnancy.

Since the bone marrow and the intestinal mucosa have an increased folic acid requirement because of a high cell proliferation rate, patients with hematological diseases, especially those with increased erythropoiesis, may not be able to meet their increased folic acid requirement from their dietary intake.

Disturbances in the absorption of folic acid occur in both tropical sprue and gluten enteropathy. Manifest macrocytic anemia may develop in both clinical pictures. Other signs of malabsorption may also occur. Alcohol-induced folic acid deficiency may to a certain extent also be caused by malabsorption.

Diseases of the small intestine may also prevent the absorption of folic acid. The folic acid absorption test is used as a general, practical means for detecting malabsorption.

Folic Acid Absorption Test

Folic acid is absorbed in the entire small intestine, so that the substance is suitable for a global test of small-intestine absorption. Data on normal serum concentrations vary slightly from laboratory to laboratory, but do not diverge to any great extent [27].

Range for folic acid in the serum:
10 – 40 nmol/l (5 – 20 µg/ml).

Procedure: The patient is given 1 mg folic acid i. v. or i. m. per day on the 4 days preceding the examination. This serves to make up any folic acid deficiency in the tissue which could affect the absorption test and produce a false positive result (no measurable increase in the serum folic acid concentration after oral ingestion). On the day of the examination the fasting patient is given 40 µg/kg folic acid orally, and the serum folic acid concentration is determined at the following times: 0, 60, 120 minutes.

In normal patients the serum concentration rises to over 170 µmol/l (75 µg/ml).

Vitamin B_{12} Deficiency

The symptoms of vitamin B_{12} deficiency are partly hematological, partly gastroenterological. Neurological manifestations are often observed independently of the duration of vitamin B_{12} deficiency [81].

There is usually tachycardia with an enlarged heart; the liver and spleen may also be slightly enlarged. Fissures in the mucous membrane, a red tongue, anorexia, weight loss and occasional diarrhea indicate that the gastrointestinal system is involved.

It may be very difficult to classify the neurological symptoms. Irrespective of the duration of the vitamin B_{12} deficit, in extreme cases they may range from demyelinization to neuron

Table 20. Causes of vitamin B_{12} deficiency

1. Inadequate intake
   - Vegetarians (rare)
2. Malabsorption
   - Deficiency of intrinsic factor
     pernicious anemia
     gastrectomy
     congenital (extremely rare)
   - Diseases of the terminal ileum
     Sprue
     Crohn's disease
     Extensive resections
     Selective malabsorption (Imerslund syndrome-extremely rare)
   - Parasite-induced deficiencies
     Fish tapeworm
     Bacteria ("blind loop syndrome")
   - Drug-induced
     PAS, neomycin

death. The earliest neurological manifestations consist of paresthesia, but also weakness, ataxia and disturbances of fine coordination. Objectively, disturbance of deep sensibility usually occurs early and Rhomberg and Babinski are positive [81]. The CNS symptoms range from forgetfulness to severe forms of dementia or psychoses. These neurological conditions may long precede the hematological manifestations, but as a rule hematological symptoms predominate in the average patient.

The main cause of vitamin B_{12} deficiency, the so-called *pernicious anemia,* is a deficiency of intrinsic factor. It is generally accompanied by atrophy of the gastric mucosa.

The disease shows geographical clustering in Northern Europe. It is generally a disease affecting the elderly beyond the age of 60; it is less common in children younger than 10 years old. It is found with striking frequency in black patients.

The current view about the pathogenesis of pernicious anemia is that it is produced by an autoimmune process directed against the parietal cells of the stomach. It is therefore most marked in patients with clinical pictures attributed to autoimmune diseases, such as immune hyperthyroidism, myxedema, idiopathic adrenal insufficiency, vitiligo and hypoparathyroidism. Antibodies against parietal cells can be detected in 90% of patients with pernicious anemia. The detection of these antibodies does not however mean that the pernicious anemia is necessarily manifest. The incidence of antibodies to intrinsic factor is about 60%.

Given the pathological mechanism involved, hypoacidity or anacidity is the rule, patients often have gastric polyps, and the incidence of stomach cancer doubles that in the normal population. If the source of the intrinsic factor is destroyed – such as by total gastrectomy or by extensive destruction of the gastric mucosa (for example by corrosion) – megaloblastic anemia may develop.

It should also not be forgotten that a number of bacteria in the intestinal flora require vitamin B_{12}. Deficiency syndromes may thus develop after anatomical lesions as a result of massive bacterial proliferation. Deficiency symptoms may also occur as a result of strictures, diverticula and the blind loop syndrome. They may also occur with pseudo obstruction in diabetes mellitus as a result of amyloid deposits, or in scleroderma. Vitamin B_{12}-deficiency anemia is also known to occur as a result of tropical sprue and the fish tapeworm. Most of these clinical pictures are also accompanied by malabsorption syndromes, often with steatorrhea.

Regional enteritis, Whipple's disease and tuberculosis may be accompanied by disturbances of vitamin B_{12} absorption. This also applies to chronic pancreatitis, in rare instances to Zollinger-Ellison syndrome and segmental diseases of the ileum [114].

Defects of absorption of vitamin B_{12} used to be detected by the Schilling Test. This test has been replaced by determination of parietal cell antibodies and antibodies against intrinsic factor.

Hereditary megaloblastic anemia is extremely rare; it is caused by congenital disturbances of orotic acid metabolism or, in Lesch-Nyhan syndrome, by the disturbance of enzymes involved in folic acid metabolism.

Table 21. Antibody-induced hemolytic anemia

1. Warm antibodies
   - Idiopathic
   - Lymphomas
   - SLE
   - Drugs
   - Neoplasms (rare)
2. Cold antibodies
   - Cold agglutinins
     Infections (generally acute)
     Lymphoma
     Idiopathic
   - Paroxysmal cold hemoglobinuria
3. Alloantibodies
   - Blood transfusions
   - Pregnancies

Normocytic Anemia

Normocytic anemia generally occurs during acute blood loss, in hemolysis and as a result of renal failure or endocrine disturbances.

Besides the formal pathological classification of anemia into microcytic, macrocytic and normocytic, differentiation by origin has now become established, especially in disturbances of erythropoiesis. The hemolytic anemias (cell trauma, membrane abnormality), enzyme disturbances (glucose-6-phosphate-dehydrogenase defect) and disturbances of hemoglobin synthesis have become clinically the most important.

Extracorpuscular Hemolytic Anemias

Hemolytic anemia is generally an acquired autoimmune hemolytic anemia. A common form of differentiation is based on the thermal behavior of the antibodies, as warm or cold antibodies.

The most common clinical pictures of symptomatic hemolytic anemia are summarized in Table 21.

In the detection of hemolysis, the determination of haptoglobin and LDH in particular have proved to be diagnostically useful tests. After the occurrence of intravascular hemolysis the haptoglobin concentration drops rapidly. This is attributable to the very short half-life of the haptoglobin-hemoglobin complex of only about 8 minutes. In its function as a transport (and acutephase) protein it binds intravascular, free hemoglobin and transports it extremely rapidly to the reticulo-endothelial system for degradation. The hemoglobin is metabolized there.

Haptoglobin is therefore eminently suitable for the detection of hemolysis, i.e., for the diagnosis and assessment of the course of hemolytic diseases. Sharply decreased haptoglobin levels indicate intravascular hemolysis which may have immunohemolytic, microangiopathic, mechanical, drug (G-6-P-dehydrogenase deficiency) or infectious causes (e.g., malaria).

Extravascular hemolysis (e.g., ineffective erythropoiesis, hypersplenism), on the other hand, shows a drop in haptoglobin only in hemolytic crises.

Reduced haptoglobin levels may also be congenital (albeit rarely in Europe). They may also be observed in other, nonhemolytic diseases, e.g. in liver diseases and in malabsorption syndrome.

Since the LDH concentration in the erythrocytes is about 360 times higher than in the plasma, with hemolytic processes there is a rise in LDH. The LDH increase stands in direct relationship

Table 22. Mechanically induced forms of hemolytic anemia

1. Microangiopathies
   - Splenomegaly
   - Hemolytic-uremic syndrome (HUS)
   - Thrombotic-thrombocytopenic purpura (TTP)
   - Disseminated intravascular coagulopathy (DIC)
   - Cirrhosis of the liver
   - Eclampsia
2. Prosthetic heart valves
3. Extracorporeal pump systems
   - Hemodialysis
   - Hemofiltration
   - Extracorporeal oxygenation

to the erythrocyte destruction. A particularly large rise in LDH can be observed in hemolytic crises. Hemolytic anemia caused by a circulatory trauma is characterized by the occurrence of burr and helmet cells. The most important clinical occurrences are listed in Table 22.

Corpuscular Anemias

The most important of the enzyme defects is glucose-6-phosphate dehydrogenase deficiency with all its genetically fixed variants, of which favism is now clinically the best known form.

The hemoglobinopathy that has attained most importance is sickle-cell anemia in all its variants; M-hemoglobin is also worthy of mention as the cause of familial cyanosis. The hemoglobinopathies also include all variants of thalassemia, a disorder which is gaining importance with the increasing mobility of the world's population. These hemoglobinopathies generally present a variable morphological picture with target cells. A clear diagnosis can be made only by hemoglobin electrophoresis or by high-pressure liquid chromatography (HPLC).

All forms of hemolytic anemia are characterized by a greater folic acid requirement because of the increased cell and iron turnover.

Deficiencies in the Cofactors of Erythropoiesis

Deficiencies in vitamin B_{12}, folic acid and erythropoietin have been found to be crucial factors in non-iron-deficiency-induced forms of anemia.

A initial diagnosis can be made with a high degree of accuracy by recording the patient's history or from knowledge of the primary disease. Given the known interaction between vitamin B_{12} and folic acid, the determination of these two cofactors by immunoassay should now be standard clinical practice.

Deficiency in folic acid or vitamin B_{12} is the main feature of diseases accompanied by macrocytic anemia.

Sternal puncture or bone biopsies also offer clear histological and morphological pictures.

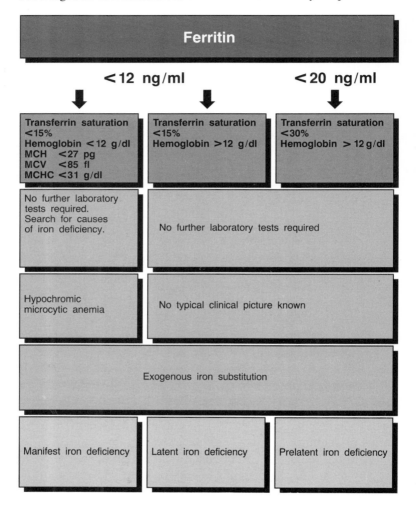

Fig. 29. Diagnostic strategy in disturbances of iron metabolism

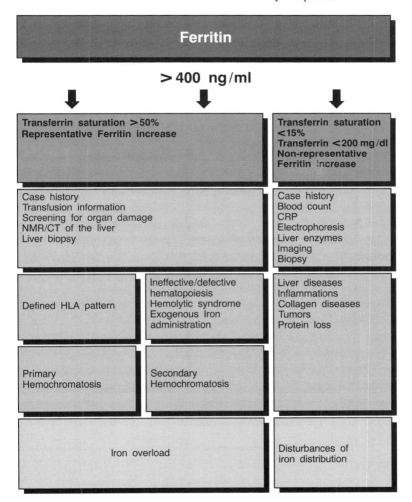

Ferritin

> 400 ng/ml

Transferrin saturation >50%
Representative Ferritin increase

Transferrin saturation <15%
Transferrin <200 mg/dl
Non-representative Ferritin increase

Case history
Transfusion information
Screening for organ damage
NMR/CT of the liver
Liver biopsy

Case history
Blood count
CRP
Electrophoresis
Liver enzymes
Imaging
Biopsy

Defined HLA pattern

Ineffective/defective hematopoiesis
Hemolytic syndrome
Exogenous Iron administration

Liver diseases
Inflammations
Collagen diseases
Tumors
Protein loss

Primary Hemochromatosis

Secondary Hemochromatosis

Iron overload

Disturbances of iron distribution

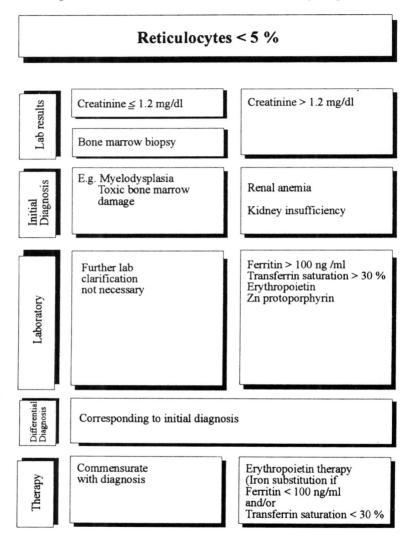

Reticulocytes < 5 %

Lab results

Creatinine $\leq$ 1.2 mg/dl

Bone marrow biopsy

Creatinine > 1.2 mg/dl

Initial Diagnosis

E.g. Myelodysplasia
Toxic bone marrow
damage

Renal anemia

Kidney insufficiency

Laboratory

Further lab
clarification
not necessary

Ferritin > 100 ng /ml
Transferrin saturation > 30 %
Erythropoietin
Zn protoporphyrin

Differential Diagnosis

Corresponding to initial diagnosis

Therapy

Commensurate
with diagnosis

Erythropoietin therapy
(Iron substitution if
Ferritin < 100 ng/ml
and/or
Transferrin saturation < 30 %

Fig. 30. Normocytic forms of anemia

Reticulocytes > 15 %

Haptoglobin > 50 mg/dl LDH < 210 U/l Bilirubin < 1 mg/dl (Free hemoglobin ⊥)	Haptoglobin < 50 mg/dl LDH > 210 U/l Bilirubin > 1 mg/dl (Free hemoglobin ↑)
Blood loss	Hemolysis

Further lab
clarification
not necessary

Erythrocyte morphology

Characteristic forms	Uncharacteristic forms
Hb-electrophoresis Osmotic resistance Erythroc. enzymes	Coombs test / \ positive negative

Corresponding to
initial diagnosis

e.g. Thalesamia Mechanic Hemolysis Spherocytosis	positive: Auto- immun- hemo- lytic anemia	negative: Toxic hemo- lysis

Blood transfusion Regular monitoring of ferritin	Therapy of underlying illness Avoidance of noxae

Table 23. Deficiencies in the cofactors of erythropoiesis

Microcytic anemia	Macrocytic anemia	Normocytic anemia
Iron metabolism disturbances	Folic acid deficiency	Renal anemia (erythropoietin deficiency)
Hemoglobinopathies	B_{12} deficiency Drug-induced Metabolic disease Uncertain origin	Hemolytic anemia Hemoglobinopathies
		Bone-marrow diseases Toxic bone marrow damage

In the differential diagnosis of macrocytic anemia, an elevated level of LDH with simultaneous reticulocytosis and hyperbilirubinemia (both to be interpreted as hyperregeneratory anemia) directs attention to a vitamin B_{12} deficit. Macrocytic anemia without these components makes a genuine folic acid deficiency likely (pregnancy, alcohol).

Normocytic forms of anemia draw attention to the hemolytic component of erythrocyte destruction, with haptoglobin playing the crucial role as the key to diagnosis. Erythrocyte morphology provides a means to exclude mechanical hemolysis or to look for hemoglobinopathy (Hb electrophoresis) or an enzyme defect.

Proof of impaired renal function makes it likely that the most important deficiency of a cofactor in Hb synthesis is present, a deficiency in erythropoietin.

The determination of erythropoietin which can now be performed by immunoassay at least forms a good base for a prognosis of response to treatment. Before giving any treatment with erythropoietin, it is important to determine the iron depots, since otherwise action by the parenterally administered erythropoietin, which is today genetically engineered, is impossible.

In summary it can be said that, given adequate iron depots, normocytic forms of anemia with normal or reduced reticulocyte counts (= disturbance of erythrocyte production) justify looking for EPO deficiency.

Therapy of Anemias

Anemias are a worldwide problem. Severe anemia affects mainly older men and women. The WHO defines anemia as a hemoglobin concentration of less than 12 g/dl in women and less than 13 g/dl in men (World Health Organization. Nutritional Anemias. Technical Reports Series 1992; 503). According to these criteria 10 to 20 percent of women and 6 to 30 percent of men above the age of 65 years are anemic.

Therapy of Iron Deficiency

Oral Administration of Iron

Oral replacement is always indicated in iron deficiency, which cannot be curid by taking in iron in the diet. In spite of various pharmaceutical formulations, the tolerability of oral iron preparations varies a great deal, so that each drug has to be monitored very carefully with regard to patient compliance.

The gold standard of therapy is still iron sulfate, which is divided into 3 daily doses. Taken on an empty stomach an iron absorption of 10-20 mg iron per day can be achieved. A significant rise in the hematocrit can be expected within 3 weeks (Table 24).

A normal red blood count (RBC) can generally be expected after 2 months but iron therapy should be continued for a further 3-6 months after reaching a normal level in order to fill the body's iron stores.

If, after two months of oral iron administration, no improvement is seen in the red blood count and diagnosis of iron deficiency anemia has been established, the main reason for a lack of improvement is that the medication has been taken irregularly or not at all. In rare cases, there are problems of absorption

Therapy of Anemias

Table 24. Recommended doses for the most common oral iron preparations

		Recommended dose
Ferrous sulfate	105 mg Fe^{2+}	Once daily
Ferrous fumarate	308 mg Fe-fumarate	Once daily
	$\cong$ 100 mg Fe^{2+}	
Ferrous gluconate	200 mg Fe-gluconate	3 x 2 tablets daily
	$\cong$ approx. 30 mg Fe^{2+}	
	625 mg Fe-gluconate	1-2 tablets daily
	$\cong$ 80 mg Fe^{2+} / ascorbic acid	

which can be excluded by the iron absorption test. If this is not the case, and it is established that the medication has been taken regularly, the diagnosis will have to be reviewed or a further search for occult blood losses should be carried out.

Parenteral Administration of Iron

The indications for i.v. iron administration are:

1. poor iron absorption
2. gastrointestinal disorders
3. the inability to mobilize adequately large iron stores already present
4. intolerance of oral iron administration.

Before administering iron parenterally, it is advisable to carry out an approximate calculation of the iron requirement and to administer it taking the iron reserves into account (Table 25).

Of the preparations available (iron dextran compounds, iron saccharate, iron gluconate, iron ascorbate, iron citrate and mixed preparations), iron saccharate has proved to be the most popular in Europe for parenteral administration (Table 26).

The iron saccharate complex has the advantage that it is not filtered through the glomeruli (molecular weight 43,000 D), is therefore not excreted renally and consequently cannot cause a tubulotoxic effect.

Table 25. Parenteral iron administration. Calculation of total dose required

Total amount of iron (g) = [Hb deficit x Blood volume x iron reserve in Hb] + Iron reserve in Depots		
Example:	Adult (male)	
	BW (body weight):	70 kg
	Blood volume:	0.069 l/kg x BW
	Hb (measured):	90 g/l
	Hb (target)	130 g/l
	Hb (deficit):	40 g/l
	Iron reserve in Hb:	3.4 mg Fe/g Hb
	Iron reserve in depots:	0.5 g (calculated by Ferritin)

Total iron dose required = [40 x 0.069 x 70 x 3.4 x 10^{-3}] + 0.5 = 0.7 + 0.5 = 1.2 (g)

Furthermore, the substance is characterized by its low potential for triggering an anaphylactic shock. However, it releases iron in the liver and from the complex and therefore hepatotoxicity should be watched for as a side effect. The table below shows the doses of iron per hemodialysis recommended as safe by the manufacturers for iron saccharate and iron gluconate.

Whereas in Europe it is customary to administer the total amount of iron in divided doses, in the United States the total dose is usually administered by intravenous infusion over a time period of 4-6 hours after giving a test dose.

The total dose for remedying a manifest iron deficiency anemia is generally between 1.5 and 2 g iron administered parenterally. In this dose, the depot iron is taken to be approximately 1.0 g.

Megaloblastic and macrocytic anemias as well as iron distribution disturbances, with or without iron deficiency, require somewhat more complex therapy.

Table 26. Parenteral iron supplementation

	Iron saccharate	Iron gluconate
< 100 Ferritin (ng/ml)	40 mg/HD*	62.5 mg/HD*
> 100 Ferritin (ng/ml)	10 mg/HD	10 mg/HD

Manufacturer's data for contents/bottle; HD = hemodialysis

Side-effects and Hazards of Iron Therapy

Oral administration of iron sulfate is regarded as standard for the therapy of iron deficiency. It is known that iron (II) salts are absorbed three times better than iron (III) salts; this discrepancy is even greater when higher doses are administered. The iron salt used has little influence on the bioavailability, since sulfate, fumarate, succinate and gluconate are absorbed approximately to the same rate and extent.

The quantity of absorbed iron is primarily dependent upon the quantity of iron and the total iron salt content in the individual forms administered. It is important that the tablets dissolve rapidly in the stomach. Although enteric coated tablets are still sold, they are quite unsuitable for oral therapy. Of the so-called absorption-enhancing substances, only ascorbic acid at a dosage of 200 mg or more has proved to be useful. It must be pointed out, however, that increased uptake is also associated with a significant rise in side-effects.

Intolerance to oral iron administration is dependent upon two factors:
1. the quantity of soluble iron in the upper gastrointestinal tract and
2. psychological factors.

Side-effects include heartburn, nausea, flatulence, constipation and diarrhea.

In order to avoid these difficulties it is advisable to start therapy with a small dosage and then gradually increase it. In approximately 25% of the patients, side-effects occur when a daily dosage of 200 mg iron is given in the form of three equally divided doses. A rise in the side-effect rate to about 40% is observed in test persons when the orally administered iron dosage is doubled. The occurrence of heartburn, constipation or diarrhea is not dependent on the administered dose.

As the oral absorption of iron in healthy persons is strictly regulated, it is virtually impossible to bring about symptoms of metal intoxication by excessive oral administration of iron to adults. Should this nevertheless occur, then hemochromatosis should be looked for. Fatalities in adults following oral administration of iron are generally the result of suicidal intent.

As has been shown by Fairbanks and Bothwell, the situation is different in children, particularly small children in the second year of life. A dose of just 1 or 2 g of iron can be fatal, although in the known cases of unintentional iron intake the doses were over 2 g (generally around 10 g). Symptoms of iron intoxication can occur within 30 min but may also not develop until several hours have elapsed. They consist of cramp-like abdominal pain, diarrhea and vomiting of brown or blood-stained gastric juice. The patients become pale or cyanotic, tired, confused, show incipient hyperventilation as a result of metabolic acidosis and die of cardiovascular failur [80].

Intravenous administration of iron is indicated above all in cases of functional iron deficiency.

During intravenous administration, intolerance reactions (immediately during or after intravenous administration) can occur. Undesired long-term side-effects in various systems of the body have also been described. Accordingly, intravenous iron therapy should only be carried out with strict adherence to the indications.

Immediate reactions include malaise, fever, acute generalized lymph adenopathy, joint pains, urticaria and occasionally exacerbation of symptoms in patients with rheumatoid arthritis. These fairly harmless but unpleasant adverse reactions differ from the rare but feared anaphylactic reactions which can be fatal despite immediate therapy. Such reactions with fatal outcome have been reported occasionally particularly for iron dextran. These occurrences necessitate very strict indications for i.v. therapy [17].

There is confirmed evidence that infections, cardiovascular diseases and carcinogenesis can be influenced by the intravenous administration of iron.

Infections: There is a close relationship between the availability of iron and the virulence of bacterial infections. This can be explained by the fact that iron is a precondition for the multiplication of bacteria in the infected body. Excessive iron can therefore increase the risk of infection. It has already been shown in human and animal studies that the intravenous administration of iron during infection causes deterioration of the clinical picture. It has in the meantime been shown that hydroxyl radicals, which are formed during iron therapy, are responsible for the negative effects of iron. In other words, iron deficiency hinders bacterial growth but also hinders adequate defense against infection in the affected organism. Particularly in dialysis patients or patients with end-stage renal disease, intravenous iron therapy can negatively influence not only the activity of the phagocytes, but also that of the T- and B-lymphocytes [97].

In patients with *malignoma*, iron therapy is clearly indicated when iron deficiency exists. However, these patients frequently suffer from ACD in which it is known that functional iron is depressed even though the iron reserves are in the normal or elevated range. Administration of iron when not indicated can not only have a detrimental effect on various organ systems of the sick person, but may also contribute to increased proliferation of neoplastic cells. Various studies have demonstrated that high transferrin saturation is associated with an elevated risk of carcinoma in general and of cancer of the lungs and colon in particular [125].

In a meta-analysis on almost 20,000 patients carried out between 1982 and 1994 it was shown that perioperative blood transfusions had a negative effect with regard to the recurrence of malignomas, increasing the risk to 37%.

In a study comparing the relative cancer risk in blood donors and non-donors, there was a significant increase in the relative risk of non-donors for developing carcinoma [74].

Recently, knowledge has grown that iron plays an increasing role in the pathogenesis of *cardiovascular disease*. The hypothesis that iron depletion has a protective action against coronary heart disease was advanced as early as 1981 [8] to explain the striking difference between the sexes regarding the incidence of coronary heart disease. It is a fact that the virtual absence of myocardial infarction in women of child-bearing age is associated with low-depot iron levels. It is also striking that after cessation of the menstrual loss of iron there is a rapid rise in the number of cases of coronary heart disease [127].

The importance of iron in atherogenesis has been demonstrated by a number of studies. One of the most recent studies showed that serum ferritin values above 50 ng/ml lead to a clear increase in atherosclerosis of the carotids in both men and women [73].

The promotion of atherogenesis during chronic intravenous iron therapy, as in hemodialysis patients, has led to considerations on the simultaneous use of erythropoietin and desferrioxamine in order to mobilize the iron depots and thus make intravenous administration of iron unnecessary. The difficulty associated with this therapy concept lies in the fact that the mobilization of depot iron cannot be predicted [9].

In the light of the aspects discussed here – namely the influence of iron on infectious disease, carcinogenesis and the development of atherosclerosis – it becomes necessary to abandon the view that more or less any quantity of stored iron is harmless provided it does not represent massive overload [9]. Every form of iron therapy therefore requires careful monitoring. Considering the aspects discussed here it should be reconsidered whether the achievement of so-called normal values for hematocrit and hemoglobin is always the right target to aim for.

Therapy of Iron Distribution Disorders

Anemia of Chronic Disease (ACD)

Anemias due to chronic pathological processes (ACD) are the result of a multifactorial process in which activation of the immune and inflammatory systems play an important role.

Therapy should be aimed primarily at healing or positively influencing the underlying disease as far as possible.

Rheumatoid Arthritis (RA)

Influencing of the inflammatory symptomatology of RA has become possible recently via therapy with monoclonal antibodies. Infliximab has been used as an antibody against the receptor of the tumor necrosis factor, TNF-α. Another possibility is the administration of a TNF-α-receptor fusion protein, Etanercept, which is reported to be easier to control.

The long-term effects of both therapeutic possibilities cannot yet be assessed, although lymphoma neogenesis must be feared from both [118] [Fig. 31].

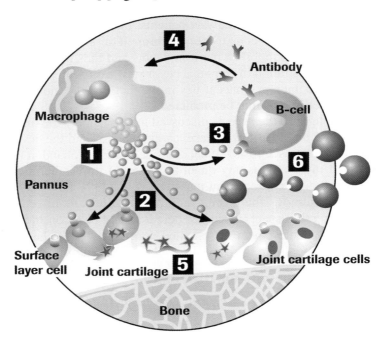

Fig. 31. Blockage of inflammation courses in the joints
1. Macrophages in the synovial fluid excrete TNF-α. **2.** TNF releases collagenases and other metallproteinases that play a significant role in the destruction of cartilage. Cell infiltration cause the synovial membrane to thicken (formation of Pannus). **3.** TNF stimulates B-cells to produce antibodies. **4.** The antibodies initiate in the macrophages the synthesis of additional TNF. **5.** The metallproteinases attack the joint cartilage and destroy bone cells. **6.** Tumor necrosis factor-(TNF-) blocking antibodies neutralize raised levels of TNF.

The use of anti-inflammatory substances such as non-steroidal anti-rheumatics, glucocorticoids, antimetabolites (methotrexate), and immunosuppressants has been established for years to treat chronic polyarthritis. Inhibition of tumor necrosis factor alpha (TNF-α) is a new therapeutic concept. TNF-α occurs at the beginning of a cascade of cytokines that eventually lead to inflammation and tissue destruction.

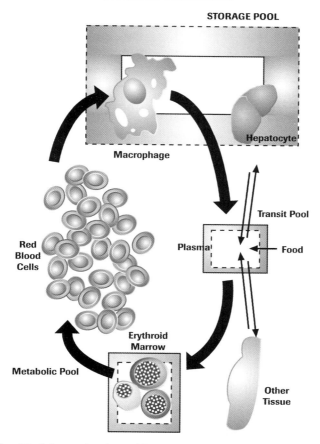

Fig. 32. Schematic view of iron metabolism. Metabolic pool – storage pool – transit pool

Under EPO / Iron - Therapy

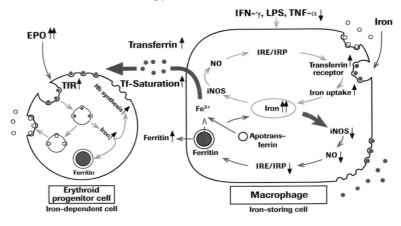

Fig. 33. Model of the autoregulatory loop between iron metabolism and the NO/NOS pathway in activated monocytes/macrophages and supply of an iron-dependent cell [140, 142]

Abbreviations:

IFN-γ, interferon γ; iNOS, induced nitric oxide synthase; IRE, iron-responsive element; IRE/IRP, high affinity binding of iron-regulatory protein (IRP) to IREs; LPS, lipopolysaccharide; TNF-α, tumor necrosis factor-α; $\uparrow$ and $\downarrow$ indicate increase or decrease of cellular responses, respectively.

Explanation of signs: ‿ Transferrin receptor,
• iron carrying transferrin;
○ apotransferrin;
⊙ ferritin.

Iron stored as ferritin within an iron-storing cell is released and bound to apotransferrin, followed by its transport to the iron-dependent cell. The cytoplasmic membrane contains transferrin receptors to which the iron-carrying transferrin binds. The endosome migrates into the cytoplasm where it releases iron. The free iron is either used as functional iron or is stored as ferritin. The endosome returns to the cytoplasmic membrane and apotransferrin is released into the extracellular space.

Table 27. EPO/i.v. iron in the treatment of ACD and DA

Correction of ACD and DA		Correction of disease activity (DA)	
EPO	50–150 IU/kg/week	EPO	50–70 IU/kg/week
i.v. iron	30-120 mg/week	i.v. iron	0–90 mg/week
Target Hb	10-12 g/dl	Target Hb	10-12 g/dl
Target ferritin	100–400 µg/l	Target ferritin	100–400 µg/l
Target s-Transferrin-		Target transferrin-	
Receptor (s-TfR)	1–3 mg/l	Saturation (TfS)	15–45%
		(TfS will be replaced by TfR in future)	
		Target s-Transferrin Receptor (s-TfR) 1– 3 mg/l	
		Target-CRP	< 5 mg/l
		ACR -Index	

Period of correction 6–12 weeks

ACD	= Anemia of chronic disease
DA	= Disease activity
TfS	= Transferrin saturation
s-TfR	= soluble-Transferrin receptor
Hb	= Hemoglobin
ACR Index	= Index of the American College of Rheumatology

Iron metabolism in monocytes/macrophages plays an especially significant role in chronic disease. The organism uses iron metabolism in the inflammatory and anti-neoplastic defense system. It draws iron from microorganisms and neoplastic cells and stores it in reticuloendothelial systems. This is characterized by the development of normochromic, normocytic anemia (ACD = Anemias of Chronic Disease). This type of anemia is caused by all types of inflammation (rheumatoid arthritis, malignant growths, or trauma). Due to various cytokines, erythropoiesis is compromised primarily at the CFU-E level in this process.

TNF-α (tumor necrosis factor-α) induces stroma cells to form inhibitory IFN-β (interferon), thereby indirectly suppressing the formation of CFU-E.

IL-1 (interleukin) induces the IFN-γ synthesis of T-cells. IFN-γ also suppresses CFU-E.

Table 28. Biochemical background for EPO/Iron combination therapy

	Erythroid cells	Reticuloendothelial system (e.g., macrophages)
EPO ↑ = EPO treatment	• stimulates proliferation of bone marrow erythroid cells	• upregulates transferrin receptor expression
	• upregulates TfR expression	• upregulates transferrin expression
"Free Iron" ↑ = i.v. iron treatment	• stimulates Hb synthesis	• inhibits NOS and NO production
		• upregulates ferritin expression
		• inhibits IFN-γ and TNF-α production

IFN-γ = Interferon-γ
TnF-α = Tumor necrosis factor α
NO   = Nitric oxide
NOS   = Nitric oxide synthesis

Monocytes/macrophages play an important role in erythropoiesis in bone marrow.

The progenitor cells of the red line proliferate and differentiate only under optimal local conditions.

The blood islands in bone marrow consist of a centrally located macrophage surrounded by small cells of the erythroid and myeloid line. The surrounding cells also comprise endothelial cells, fat cells, reticuloepithelial cells, and fibroblasts.

Erythropoietin (EPO) is the most important and specific erythropoiesis-stimulating factor. It acts on early progenitor cells up to the maturation levels after the erythroblast. Without EPO, erythroid differentiation does not progress past the level of burst forming units (BFU-E).

Iron and erythropoietin therapy in patients with *autoimmune diseases* (such as rheumatoid arthritis) can be assessed as promising [18, 94], as in addition to improving the anemia, the

Table 29. Recommendations for iron replacement therapy in ACD patients receiving rhEPO therapy

Diagnostic Parameter	Target Values	Frequency of Determination
Hematological parameters		
Hemoglobin	10–12 g/dl	
Hematocrit	30–36 %	monthly
Reticulocytes	10–15 ‰	
Folate	> 20 ng/ml	every 6 months
Vitamin B_{12}	> 2 ng/ml	during treatment
Iron parameters		
Ferritin (F)	100–400 ng/ml	At beginning of correction
Transferrin saturation	15–45 %	phase and 3 weeks after end
Hypochromic erythrocytes	< 10 %	of correction phase
Soluble transferrin receptor (s-TfR)	1-3 mg/l	At end of correction phase and
TfR/log F		every three months after end
CRP	< 5 mg/l	of correction phase

After commencing with rhEPO therapy and approx. 3 weeks after the end of the correction phase with i.v. iron, all hematological parameters and iron parameters should be determined.

previously described inhibiting effect of iron on cytokine action and macrophage-induced cytotoxicity has a favorable influence.

As under erythropoietin administration the transferrin receptor on erythroid precursor cells is upregulated, the sequential administration of erythropoietin and iron (at intervals of 48 hours) should be discussed. It is possible that negative reactions with regard to the immune response can be reduced [146].

The patients were treated with 150 IU rhEPO per kg body weight twice weekly over a period of 12 weeks. Where there was a functional iron deficit, the patients were additionally given 200 mg Fe^{3+}-sucrose weekly i.v.

All patients showed normalization of Hb concentration and quality of life as measured by various parameters such as multidimensional assessment of fatigue (MAF) and muscle strength index (MSI). Laboratory parameters for the activity of rheumatoid arthritis and rheumatoid arthritis disease activity index (RADAI) also showed a clear improvement during erythropoietin therapy. Upon cessation of therapy after the 12-week period there was – as expected – a decrease in the improvement achieved.

The doses of erythropoietin and iron necessary for correction and maintenance were no higher than those required for anemia resulting from chronic renal failure.

In a placebo-controlled, double-blind study by Peeters et al. [98], it was shown that in addition to compensating anemia there was, above all, regression of inflammatory disease activity in rheumatoid arthritis [99].

In order to achieve optimum management of patients treated with rhEPO in combination with intravenous iron injections, the iron balance parameters listed in Table 29 should be determined at regular intervals.

Recommendations for the treatment of anemia in RA have been updated. At the moment, virtually identical recommendations apply both to the treatment of anemia in RA (iron distribution disorder) and to anemia due to renal failure (erythropoietin deficiency and iron utilization disorder) (Table 27).

Therapy of Chronic Inflammatory Processes

As has been mentioned already, these anemias are the result of a multifactorial process in which the activation of the immunological and inflammatory systems play an important role [138].

Pretherapeutic erythropoietin levels in tumor patients seem to be of predictive value regarding the effectivity of erythropoietin therapy in any given patient: tumor anemias having an initial erythropoietin level of less than 500 mU/ml respond very well to the administration of erythropoietin [87].

Ludwig et al. [87] reported on a successful therapy regime in which a rise in the hemoglobin concentration of 0.5 g/dl and a reduction in the erythropoietin concentration to less than 100 mU/ml was observed after 2 weeks. A decrease in the serum ferritin level was also interpreted as being a positive sign of therapeutic success. The disease modifying drugs used in the context of the therapy of rheumatic diseases as well as successful tumor therapy may also play a role.

A response to erythropoietin therapy can be expected after 4–6 weeks on average, whereby one should note that not all tumors respond in the same favorable manner and the choice of chemotherapy is of importance.

Clinical experience shows that a dosage of 150 U/kg body weight/3 x weekly leads to the following response rates: multiple myeloma (approx. 82%), breast carcinomas (approx. 43%), colon carcinomas (approx. 52%). The response rates for patients suffering from myelodysplastic syndrome is in contrast low and is less than 10% [88]. The therapy of anemias of inflammation is remarkably similar to that for uremia. Inadequate erythropoietin secretion seems to warrant the use of recombinant rhEPO to correct the anemia when functional iron deficiency is rectified in time by adequate iron replacement. The recommended EPO dose is 150 U/kg of body weight administered subcutaneously twice weekly. Initial therapeutic results are very encouraging because of the fact that concomitant anemia in highly active rheumatoid arthritis can also be successfully treated by erythropoietin substitution. After eradicating the functional iron deficiency by administering iron parenterally, a normalization of the hemoglobin concentration is then possible in ACD by administering erythropoietin. Iron (III) sucrose complex is recommended for intravenous iron therapy.

The important aspect of erythropoietin and i.v. iron substitution therapy in ACD in the context to rheumatoid arthritis was published recently by Kessler et al. [72] in the Frankfurt ACD study. This is in agreement with the results of Weiss et al. [138].

To guarantee optimal patient care for patients receiving rhEPO in combination with i.v. Fe (III) injections, body iron store parameters (see Table 29) should be determined at regu-

lar intervals during both the corrective phase and the maintenance phase.

Therapy of Iron Utilization Disorders

Erythropoietin Deficiency, Anemia in Renal Failure

The development and introduction of recombinant human erythropoietin has made the causal therapy of renal anemia possible
[46, 115].
Remarkably, uremic anemia is well tolerated by patients and
hemoglobin values up to 5 g/dl are well tolerated without side effects. In most patients the reticulocyte count is low and the survival time of blood cells is only moderately decreased. Anemia is
thus the result of a massively disturbed erythrocyte production in
the bone marrow.

The difficulty of successful therapy of renal anemia is however to correct the transport iron deficiency and avoid a significant
iron overload. Transferrin saturation should be significantly more
than 20% and storage iron levels should exceed 100 ng/ml of ferritin, if absolute or functional iron deficiency as the cause of an inadequate therapeutic response to recombinant erythropoietin
(rhEPO) is to be excluded.

Low serum ferritin values (less than 100 ng/ml) in patients with
uremia signify an absolute iron deficiency, high ferritin values,
however, do not completely exclude functional iron deficiency.

Functional iron deficiency is characterized by non-pathological (100-300 ng/ml ferritin in women, 100-400 ng/ml ferritin in
men) or elevated ferritin values as well as reduced transferrin saturation values (less than 20%).

Criteria for a sufficient supply of iron are a ferritin level of
at least 100 ng/ml and a transferrin saturation of more than 20%.
The soluble transferrin receptor concentration should be equal
to or less than 3 mg/l (values are dependent on the method
used).

If dialysis patients do not meet these criteria, then 10 mg of
iron per dialysis should be administered after replenishing the

iron depot to a ferritin level of 100 ng/ml. In non-dialysis patients oral iron replacement may be adequate (100 to 300 mg/day). The therapeutic aim is to increase the hemoglobin concentration to 10-12 g/dl. The total iron requirement can be estimated using the following formula:

Estimation of Iron requirement

Iron requirement (g) = 0,15 x (Hb_1 – Hb_0)
Hb_1 is the target hemoglobin concentration in g/dl
Hb_0 is the initial hemoglobin concentration in g/dl

The therapeutic targets are listed in Table 30.

Ferritin values of over 400 ng/ml should be avoided in the long term on account of the concomitant danger of iron deposits forming outside the reticuloendothelial system.

If values exceed this threshold during intravenous therapy, then a pause in the therapy for a period of 3 months should be considered but erythropoietin treatment should be continued. The danger of iron overload in the context of parenteral substitution therapy adapted to iron losses of approximately 2000 mg per annum can be considered to be low for hemodialysis patients. In the maintenance phase a low-dose, high-frequency administration of iron (10 to a maximum of 20 mg iron saccharate per hemodialysis) is currently preferred.

Table 30. Objectives for the iron metabolism of dialysis patients undergoing i.v. iron therapy

---

- Replacement of any depot iron deficiency (rare)
  Objective: 100 ng/ml $\geq$ ferritin $\leq$ 400 ng/ml
- Treatment of a transport iron deficiency
  (frequent, due to iron mobilization disturbances)
  Objective: 15 % > transferrin saturation $\leq$ 45 %
- Avoidance of a significant iron overload
  Warning limits: Tf saturation > 45 %
  Ferritin > 400 ng/ml
  (if there are no disturbances in iron distribution)

Table 31. Recommendations for diagnosis in patients on
hemodialysis undergoing EPO therapy

Diagnostic parameter	Target values	Frequency of determination
Hematological parameters		
Hemoglobin	10-12g/dl	
Hematocrit	30-36 %	Monthly
Reticulocytes	10-15 ‰	
Folate	> 20 ng/ml	Every 6 months
Vitamin B_{12}	> 2 ng/ml	during treatment
Iron parameters		
Ferritin (F)	100-400 ng/ml	At beginning of correction
Transferrin saturation	15-45 %	phase and 3 weeks after end
Hypochromic erythrocytes		of correction phase
Soluble transferrin receptor (S-TfR)	1-3 mg/l	At end of correction phase
TfR/log F		and every three months after
CRP	< 5 mg/l	end of correction phase

After commencing with rhEPO therapy and approx. 3 weeks after the end of the
correction phase with i.v. iron, all hematological parameters and iron parameters
should be determined.

No acute phase reaction was detected in patients undergoing
dialysis who were administered iron as shown by the determination of CRP, IL-6 (interleukin-6), orosomucoid (alpha1-acid-gly-
coprotein) and SAA (serum-amyloid-A-protein).

Possible side effects of long-term iron supplementation caus-
ing ferritin values to exceed 400 mg/ml are: increased risk of
infection, elevated risk of developing carcinomas and an increased cardiovascular risk [97, 125, 127].

During rhEPO therapy with concomitant iron supplementation one should try to avoid iron-overload.

In the context of the therapy of uremic anemia, the erythropoietin doses administered should be matched to the individual
needs of the patient because the-amount required by the uremic
patient can be subject to considerable change. Provided iron re-

Table 32. Recommendations for iron replacement in dialysis patients

Diagnostic parameters	Fe deficiency	Iron status Adequate Fe stores	Fe overload
Diagnosis			
Hemoglobin		10-12 g/dl	
Hematocrit		30-36%	
Erythrocytes			
Hypochromic			
erythrocytes			
Reticulocytes		10-15‰	
Ferritin (ng/ml)	≤ 100	≥ 100	> 400 warning limit: 400
Transferrin saturation (%)	≤ 15	≥ 15	> 45
Soluble transferrin			
receptor (s-TfR)			
(mg/l)	> 5		
• Iron therapy	10-40 mg iron	0-30 mg iron	no iron
i.v./dialysis or	i.v./ dialysis		
100-300 mg iron			
orally daily			
• EPO therapy	2000 IU/patient/dialysis		

CRP
GPT
CHE

serves are sufficient it is, however, much lower than previously assumed. The erythropoietin dose can be significantly reduced in dialysis patients receiving optimized intravenous iron therapy. Hörl reported a reduction in the mean EPO dosage from 217 to 62 U/kg/week and Schäfer a reduction from 144 to 68 U/kg/week [57].

The often discussed question of whether the dosage of erythropoietin is influenced by the route of administration is best answered by pointing out that, on parenteral iron therapy, there is no

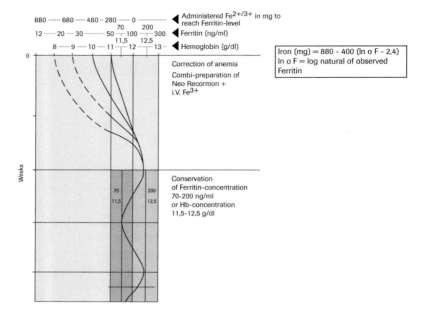

Fig. 34. Cook's equation for renal anemia. How much iron/rhEPO should be administered per dialysis to achieve a target value of 100 ng/ml ferritin and 12 g/l hemoglobin? [Cook, JD et al. (1986) Blood 687: 726-731, and Mercuriali, F. et al. (1994) Transfusion 34: 501-506]

significant difference in the amount of erythropoietin required by intravenous and by subcutaneous administration. Similar observations were made by Sunder-Plasmann and Hörl [57, 129].

Cook and coworkers as well as Mercuriali and coworkers have developed a therapeutic regimen for hemodialysis patients receiving rhEPO in which the targets are 100 ng/ml serum ferritin and a transferrin saturation of more than 20% in order to ensure provision of adequate amounts of iron without the risk of iron overload.

These recommendations are summarized in Fig. 33.

$$\text{Iron (mg)} = 880 - 400 \times (\ln \text{oF} - 2.4)$$
$$\ln \text{oF} = \log \text{ natural of observed ferritin}$$

Deficiencies in the Cofactors of Erythropoiesis

Vitamin B$_{12}$ Deficiency

The most frequent cause of B$_{12}$ deficiency is a lack of intrinsic factor, as in pernicious anemia or after a total gastrectomy. Reduced absorption in the ileum after extensive surgical resection or in Crohn's disease may also be a cause. All other causes have little practical relevance. Vitamin B$_{12}$ must be administered parenterally. On account of the neurological and neuropsychiatric syndromes, which may also occur without blood count changes, and which are only then are definitely reversible if they have been present for less than 6 months, an initial high-dose treatment regimen has become established.

This is a stepped regimen, in which 200 µg vitamin B$_{12}$ is administered intramuscularly daily during the first week of therapy, followed by one intramuscular injection per week for 1 month and then monthly administration for the rest of the patient's life.

It should be pointed out again that pernicious anemia is a life-long disease and that if the monthly treatment is interrupted, this will inevitably lead to a vitamin deficiency.

Clinical improvement is usually seen immediately after administration of vitamin B$_{12}$. Between the 5th and 7th day, if there are sufficient iron reserves, the so-called reticulocytic crisis appears and within 2 months the peripheral blood count has returned to normal.

Hypokalemia may occur in the early days of the treatment.

Folic Acid Deficiency

Low levels of folic acid in the serum or in the erythrocytes are a definite indication of folic acid deficiency.

This condition is treated by oral replacement therapy, with 1 mg folic acid being administered daily. The reaction to the replacement therapy is similar to that in B$_{12}$, deficiency, within 5 to 7 days there is an increase in the number of reticulocytes and the blood count returns to normal within 2 to 3 months.

The main cause of folic acid deficiency is an inadequate supply in the food (alcoholism, unbalanced diets, drugs). If these factors are not present in the patient's history, a B$_{12}$ deficiency should also be ruled out.

Autologous Blood Donors

It has also been demonstrated that in autologous blood donors the pre-operative administration of erythropoietin increases erythrocyte production in proportion to the dose administered.

Other Indications

Erythropoietin is now also used in the treatment of other types of anemia apart from uremic anemia, e.g. ACD, as well as in patients with AIDS [53].

The best treatment of ACD is the treatment and cure of the underlying disease. The administration of iron to patients with ACD is controversial, although the cell mediated immune effector mechanism may be weakened by the action of iron.

On the other hand erythropoietin therapy in ACD is widely used, although sometimes with low response rates. Erythropoietin is able to up-regulate TfR expression in erythroblasts and therefore affects iron balance by reducing ferritin depots and transferring them into hemoglobin.

It seems to be promising to administer erythropoietin and iron intravenously either at the same time or in sequence (iron 48 hours later) to reach a transferrin saturation > 15%. Kaltwasser suggests 2 x 150 U EPO/kg/week together with 200 mg iron-sucrose i.v./week for correction of ACD. The purpose of the iron administration is to correct the functional iron deficiency and thus also the disturbance of iron distribution in ACD. [72]

To achieve the desired hemoglobin (13 g/dl), treatment for approximately 9 weeks was necessary. There are no valid data available indicating how this beneficial effect can be maintained. In two publications the EPO doses necessary to maintain the Hb levels vary between 12.5 and 240 U/kg/Body Weight, but it is noteworthy that no iron supplements to correct functional iron deficiency were given.

The changes in lipid metabolism on erythropoietin therapy are also worthy of mention. A significant decrease in serum cholesterol has been seen [77].

Methods

The methods of determination for the blood count, the iron metabolism and for inflammation are only described in principle; the listed references allow the reader to obtain further and more detailed information. The recommended reference intervals apply only to the methods described in the respective references.

The development of new methods, the improvement of existing methods, high quality standards as well as increasing national and international standardization have resulted in an increase in the clinical sensitivity and specificity of clinical laboratory-diagnostic investigations.

The Blood Count

Complete blood count: the CBC is a basic evaluation that usually includes Hb, Hct, WBC count, WBC differential count, platelet count, a description of the blood smear relative to RBC morphology and degree of polychromatophilia, and platelet spread and architecture. An RBC count is often included, especially when calculation of RBC indices is desired.

Indications for a CBC include suspected hematologic, inflammatory, neoplastic, or infectious disease.

Anemia, erythrocytosis, leukemia, bone marrow failure, infection, inflammation, or adverse drug reactions may be detected. Blood smear examination can help detect other abnormalities (e.g. thrombocytopenia, malarial and other parasites, significant formation of rouleaux, nucleated RBCs or immature granulocytes, inclusions in RBCs or granulocytes) that may occur despite normal counts. Evaluation of the blood smear is important for assessment of RBC morphology and abnormal WBCs.

Table 33. Parameters determined in routine hematology

	Complete blood count (CBC)	Differential blood count
		3-part differential
Information on number and type of blood cells	White blood cells (WBC)	Lymphocytes / Monocytes / Granulocytes
	Red blood cells (RBC) Platelets (Plt)	**5-part differential** Lymphocytes Monocytes Neutrophils / Basophils / Eosinophils
The hemoglobin concentration as biochemical parameter	Hemoglobin (Hb)	
The volume of (red blood) cells as percentage of total blood volume	Hematocrit (Hct) [or packed cell volume (PCV)]	
Different red blood cell indices to define size and Hb content of RBCs (calculated using Hb, RBC and Hct)	Mean cell volume (MCV) Mean cell Hb (MCH) Mean cell Hb-concentration (MCHC)	

Basic Tests of Hematopoiesis

The basic investigation is the automated complete blood count which represents a profile of tests provided by hematology analyzers. The basic blood count of modern hematology analyzers consists of the following parameters:
– hemoglobin (Hb)
– white blood cell (WBC) count
– red blood cell (RBC) count
– hematocrit (HCT)
– mean cell volume of red cells (MCV)

– mean cell hemoglobin content of red cells (MCH)
– mean cell hemoglobin concentration of red cells (MCHC)
– platelet (PLT) count.

Through automated technology, the RBC count, Hb, Hct, and platelet count are available in about 30 sec. In rare cases, blood counts can also be measured by mixing a measured volume of blood with an appropriate diluent or lysing agent and counting in a chamber under the microscope. Hb can be measured colorimetrically after treatment with dilute hydrochloric acid, which permits colorimetric or spectrophotometric comparison with standards of hematin or cyanmethemoglobin, respectively. Hct can be measured by centrifuging a volume of blood and determining the percentage of RBCs relative to total blood volume. The WBC differential count is measured by staining a drop of blood on a glass slide with a metachromatic stain (e.g., Wright's) and examining it with oil immersion microscopy.

Automated Cell Counting

Automated cell counting with a hematology system using an impedance or an optical principle is now routine in many hematology laboratories. Most hematology systems use the impedance principle. In the last few years a trend towards use of optical methods (fluorescence flow cytometry) for determination of the differential blood count has been observed.

Blood specimen collection: blood is preferably collected by venipuncture, although fingertip puncture with a sterile lancet may sometimes suffice.

Ethylenediaminetetraacetic acid (EDTA) is the preferred anticoagulant for blood collection because the morphology is less distorted and platelets are better preserved. It can be added to clean test tubes, or vacuum tubes containing EDTA may be obtained commercially. Slides should be prepared within 3 to 4 h after obtaining blood, or within 1 to 2 h for platelet counts.

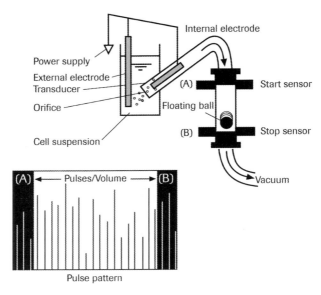

Fig. 35. Impedance principle

The Impedance Principle

EDTA blood is diluted with a defined volume of electrolyte solution and placed in a transducer chamber which is connected with a further electrolyte solution via a small orifice (50–100 µm). A constant electric current is applied between electrodes on either side of the orifice. The cell suspension is drawn through the measuring orifice by means of a vacuum. When a cell passes through the orifice it acts as non-conductor and the resistance increases. Using Ohm's law a pulse proportionate to the volume can be derived. In systems using absolute measurement (number of cells per volume) the counting volume is determined with the help of manometers. Systems using the principle of relative measurement determine the cell count per unit of time. In this case the counting rate must then be converted to the cell count per volume with the help of a calibration solution (Fig. 34).

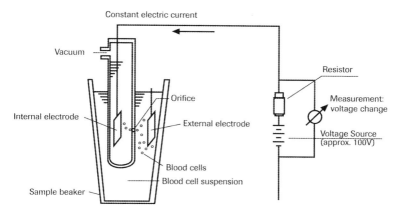

Fig. 36. Impedance principle (absolute counting) with pulse pattern produced by the measuring system; pulse counting per unit of volume

The described measuring principle for particle counting using an absolute measuring system permits the counting of red cells, white cells and platelets (Fig. 35). On account of their different concentrations, these three parameters must be counted in two different dilutions (Fig. 36). In a first dilution the white cells are analyzed after the erythrocytes have been lysed by a lysing agent. In a second, higher dilution the red cells and platelets are counted. On account of their different sizes, red cells and platelets can be differentiated from each by pulse thresholds known as discriminators. Many systems use variable thresholds, i.e. the ideal discriminators are determined for each sample measured. This prevents parts of a cell population from being cut off and therefore not included in the count.

Flow Cytometry

Flow cytometry is a measurement method for assessing particles in aqueous suspension. It is suitable for measuring single cells contained in blood and in other body fluids [124].

The procedural steps are in principle as follows:

Venous/capillary EDTA whole blood
Minimum volume: 20 µl

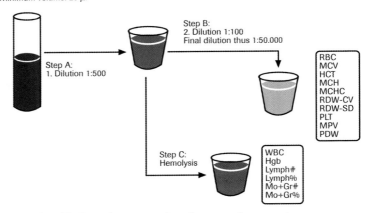

Fig. 37. Sample preparation for a semiautomatic counter

The optical system employs a semi-conductive laser. This 650 nm beam is shaped and focused onto the flow cell.

When the blood cells suspended in the diluent pass through the flow cell, the blood cells are radiated with rays from the laser beam, generating scattered light in intensities proportional to the size of the blood cells. The low-angle (1-6°) scattered light reflects cell size, and the high angle (8-20°) scattered light reflects intracellular density (nucleus size and density). The photo-diode receives these scattered lights and converts them into electrical pulses.

The cells are transported in a laminar fluid stream like pearls in a chain by using a special technique (hydrodynamic focusing) and become illuminated at the interrogation point by a light beam.

The light scattered at the interrogation point by the cell is evaluated at different angles thus defining different characteristics of the cells or particles involved. The scatter characteristics strongly depend on the wavelength of the light and the particle size.

Immunofluorescence

The fluorescence of cells or particles can be measured. Before flow cytometry cells or particles are either stained with fluo-

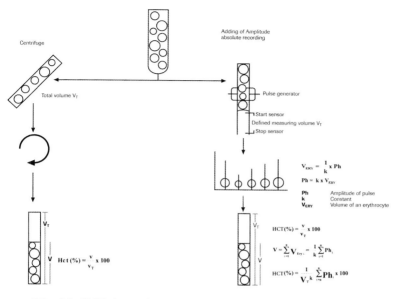

Fig. 38. HCT-determination by means of cumulative impulse amplitude adding compared with centrifugation

rochromes or labeled with fluorescence conjugated antibodies. Excitation of fluorescence is usually by an argon laser (488 nm) emitting blue-green light or a helium-neon laser (633 nm) with red light emission. The fluorochromes therefore must have their absorption maximum near these wavelengths. Thus depending on the application or staining technique used, either protein-fluorochrome conjugates such as fluorescent-labeled antibodies or affinity-bound dyes, e.g. thiazole orange, for reticulocyte RNA staining, are available [124].

Immunofluorescence, i.e. labeling by means of high affinity monoclonal antibodies which are covalently linked to a fluorescent dye and stoichiometric staining of nucleic acids are the most important staining techniques. Furthermore, there are increasing numbers of tests involving cellular function such as enzyme activities, cytokine synthesis and apoptosis.

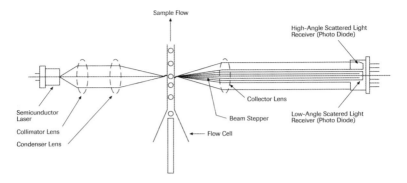

Fig. 39. Schematic illustration of a Laser-based flow cytometer

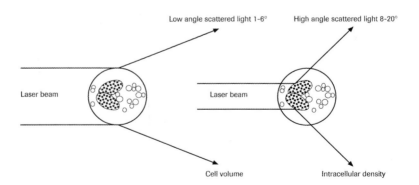

Fig. 40. Scattered light detection method
On each individual cell, 2 measurements are done:
1. Low-angle (1-6°) scattered light which reflects cell size.
2. High-angle (8-20°) scattered light which reflects intracellular
structure (nucleus size and cytoplasm density)

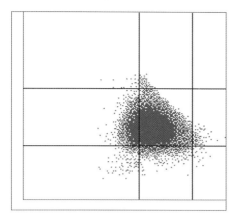

Fig. 41. Morphology of the erythrocytes (diagnosis of anemias, monitoring of therapies)

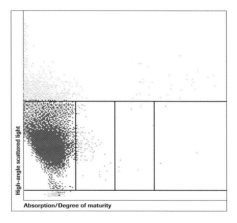

Fig. 42. Classification of reticulocytes (degree of maturity, indices)

Hemoglobin (Hb)

The hemoglobins in the blood comprise a group of hemoglobin derivatives, namely:

- Desoxyhemoglobin (HHb)
- Oxyhemoglobin (O_2Hb)
- Carboxyhemoglobin (COHb)
- Hemiglobin (Hi), also called methemoglobin (MetHb)

These hemoglobin derivatives, which are present in cell-bound form, are determined in whole blood. Free hemoglobin, that is the hemoglobin released from the erythrocytes, on the other hand, is determined in plasma.

Measurement of Hemoglobin

Photometric measurement of hemoglobin is an integral part of present-day hematology systems. The measurement is performed either with part of the leukocyte dilution, in which case the hemoglobin released by lysis of the red cells is transformed into stable derivatives and measured photometrically, or in a separate dilution with a lysing agent specially designed for hemoglobin determination. The latter procedure has the advantage that the lysing agent used is optimized for hemoglobin measurement. There is therefore no need to take into account the sensitivity of the leukocytes and the dilution ratio most appropriate for hemoglobin determination can be used. A separate hemoglobin channel with a separate hemoglobin lysing agent is subject to less interference by high leukocyte concentrations than hemoglobin photometry as part of the WBC counting.

In the past many hematology systems used a modified cyanmethemoglobin method for hemoglobin determination. This has the disadvantage that the solution contains cyanide and must therefore be disposed of as toxic waste. The introduction of a cyanide-free hemoglobin reagent has largely eliminated this problem. This reagent contains sodium lauryl sulfate as active component.

Principle of the Hemiglobincyanide Method

In solution, the Fe^{2+} of hemoglobin is oxidized to Fe^{3+} by potassium ferricyanide [$K_3Fe(CN)_6$] forming hemiglobin (Hi). This reacts with the cyanide ions (CN-) made available in the solution by potassium cyanide, forming cyanmethemoglobin

(HiCN). The absorbance of HiCN is measured at 540 nm. The hemiglobincyanide method is the reference method [132].

$$Hb(Fe^{2+}) \xrightarrow{K_3Fe\ (CN_6)} MetHb\ (Fe^{3+}) \xrightarrow{KCN} (HiCN)$$

MetHb = Methemoglobin
HiCN = Cyanmethemoglobin

Reference range [51]:

Adults:	Women	12.3-15.3 g/dl	7.6-9.5 mmol/l
	Men	14.0-17.5 g/dl	8.7-10.9 mmol/l

According to the WHO criteria a hemoglobin concentration of less than 12 g/dl in women and less than 13 g/dl in men indicates anemia. On this basis, 10 to 22 percent of women and 6 to 30 percent of men over the age of 65 years have anemia.

Hematocrit (Hct)

The hematocrit, or packed cell volume (PCV), is the ratio of the volume of red cells to the volume of whole blood in a sample of venous or capillary blood. The ratio is measured after appropriate centrifugation. In laboratory practice the hematocrit is usually expressed as a percentage.

$$Hct\ (\%) = \frac{Volume\ of\ Erythrocytes\ x\ 100}{Volume\ of\ Whole\ blood}$$

The hematocrit is a further important parameter in laboratory hematology. It is also determined automatically by many hematology systems today. Figure 36 shows a schematic comparison of pulse height summation, the method used by many hematology systems, and the centrifugal hematocrit. The cells which pass through the measuring orifice generate pulses which are proportionate to their volume. The hematocrit is obtained by summation of the individual pulses which are between an upper and lower discriminator. The result is multiplied by a constant factor which takes into account the dilution ratio. The results of the hematology analyzers are standardized against the microhematocrit method.

Microhematocrit Method

Borosilicate or soda-lime glass capillary tubes having a length of 75 mm and an internal diameter of 1.15 mm are recommended. The wall thickness should be 0.20 mm. The requirements for centrifugation are as follows:

- Microhematocrit centrifuge with a rotor radius > 8 cm
- Maximum speed should be reached within 30 sec
- Relative centrifugal force 10,000 - 15,000 x g at the periphery for 5 min without exceeding a temperature of 45°C.

The hematocrit is calculated as follows:

$$Hct = \frac{\text{Length of red cell column (mm)}}{\text{Length of red cell column plus plasma column (mm)}}$$

The microhematocrit method is the reference method [132]

Reference intervals [51]:

Women	0.35–0.47	35–47 %
Men	0.40–0.52	40–52 %

Erythrocytes

The differentiation of stem cells to erythrocytes begins at the level of the hematopoietic stem cell (CFU-GEMM). From this stage on, all successor cells of erythropoiesis have lost their ability to renew erythropoiesis.

The hematopoietic stem cell (CFU-GEMM) differentiates into the burst forming unit erythroid (BFU-E). This stage is followed by the colony forming unit erythroid (CFU-E). After various divisions, which take several days in vivo, the cells go through a process of typical morphological and functional differentiation in the process of which they lose their proliferative capacity step by step.

As the erythrocytes age, they decrease in volume and deformability and their density increases. Changes in the cell membrane lead to loss of carbohydrates on the cell surface. The normal red cell is removed from the blood stream by the reticuloendothelial system by phagocytosis after 100-120 days.

Red Cell Count (RBC)

The red cell count is a basic examination for the evaluation of disorders of erythropoiesis. For more detailed evaluation the hemoglobin concentration and the mean corpuscular volume (MCV) of the red cells and the red cell distribution width (RDW) are determined.

Reference interval:

Women	4.1-5.1
Men	4.5-5.9

Values in $10^6/\mu l$ or $10^{12}/l$

The red cell count alone is of little diagnostic value. Only the combination of this parameter with the hematocrit permits differentiation between erythrocytopenia, erythrocytosis or a normal erythrocyte count with reference to the red cell mass of the body.

RBC Indices: MCV, MCH, MCHC

Hematology analyzers calculate the following parameters from the measured red cell count and hemoglobin concentration:

- mean corpuscular volume (MCV)
- mean corpuscular hemoglobin (MCH)
- mean corpuscular hemoglobin concentration (MCHC)

The MCV, MCH and MCHC are called red cell indices and are used for the description of red cell changes and the differentiation of disturbances of erythropoiesis.

MCV = the mean cell volume of the red cell. The MCV is expressed in femtoliters (fl). Hematology analyzers either measure this parameter directly or calculate it according to the following equation:

$$MCV \ (fl) = \frac{Hematocrit \ x \ 10^3}{Red \ cells \ per \ liter}$$

MCH = the mean hemoglobin content of the red cell. The MCH is expressed in picograms (pg) and is calculated by hematology analyzers using the following equation:

$$MCH(pg) = \frac{\text{Hemoglobin concentration (g/dl)}}{\text{Red cells per liter } (10^{12}/l}$$

MCHC = the mean hemoglobin concentration of the red cells. The MCHC is expressed in g/dl of red blood cells and is calculated as follows:

$$MCHC\ (g/dl) = \frac{\text{Hemoglobin concentration (g/dl)}}{\text{Hematocrit}}$$

The *calculated parameters* MCV, MCH, MCHC are obtained by calculation from the parameters red cell concentration per liter, hemoglobin concentration and hematocrit [132].

MCV, MCH, MCHC are important for:
- the classification of anemias
- the early detection of processes which can cause anemia

Reference intervals [51]

MCV (fl)	MCH (pg)	MCHC (g/dl)
80-96	28-33	33-36

Determination of the MCV is used for the diagnostically important distinction between normocytic, microcytic and macrocytic anemias. The MCV is dependent on the hydration of the red cells and on the red cell distribution width in the plasma.

In the majority of the anemias the MCH correlates with the MCV. Microcytic anemias correspond to hypochromic anemias, normocytic to normochromic anemias.

The MCHC is a measure of the hemoglobin concentration of the circulating red cell mass. On account of the parallel behavior of the red cell volume and the hemoglobin content of the individual red cells the MCHC remains constant in many red cell changes.

The type of anemia may be indicated by the RBC indices: mean corpuscular volume (MCV), mean corpuscular Hb (MCH), and mean corpuscular Hb concentration (MCHC). RBC populations

Table 34. Classification of the anemias on the basis of
MCV, MCH and MCHC

Red cell indices	Evaluation

MCV normal
MCH normal
MCHC normal
	Normochromic, normocytic anemia:
	– non regenerative anemias, e.g.
	  chronic diseases of the kidneys,
	  endocrine disorders, maldigestion,
	  malabsorption, malignant tumors.

MCV normal MCH elevated / normal MCHC elevated / normal	Normocytic, normo/hyperchromic anemia: – hemolysis – spherocytosis (MCHC elevated)
MCV elevated MCH normal / elevated MCHC normal/decreased	– Folate or vitamin B12 deficiency anemia – Liver cirrhosis – Alcoholism
MCV reduced MCH reduced MCHC normal	– Most common form of anemia. – ACD – An underlying deficiency of iron, copper or vitamin B6 is present

are termed microcytic (MCV < 80 fl) or macrocytic (MCV > 95 fl).
The term hypochromia refers to RBC populations with MCH < 27
pg/RBC or MCHC < 30%. These quantitative relationships can
usually be recognized on a peripheral blood smear and, together
with the indices, permit a classification of anemias [132].

Automated electronic techniques directly measure Hb, RBC
count and MCV, whereas Hct, MCH, and MCHC are derived
from these data. Thus, the MCV has become the most important
RBC index in the differential diagnosis of anemias, and confidence in the derived figures (especially Hct) has declined.
Automated-flow cytometry provides a new parameter in differential diagnosis: A histogram of anisocytosis (variation in cell
size) can be automatically expressed on the coefficient of variation of the RBC volume distribution width (RDW).

Poikilocytosis (variation in shape) may also occur. RBC injury may be identified by finding RBC fragments, portions of disrupted cells (schistocytes), or evidence of significant membrane alterations from oval-shaped cells (ovalocytes) or spherocytic cells. Target cells (thin RBCs with a central dot of Hb) are RBCs with insufficient Hb or excess membrane.

Reticulocytes

Reticulocytes are a transitional form between the nucleated erythroblast and the anucleate mature erythrocyte. The reticulocyte is a very young erythrocyte which contains precipitated nucleic acids after supravital staining. For identification as a reticulocyte the cell must contain two or more clumps or blue-stained granules which must be visible microscopically without fine-focussing of the cell.

Reticulocyte Count

Determination of the reticulocyte count is used for:

- distinction between hypo-, normo- and hyperregenerative forms of anemia,
- determination of the bone marrow activity in normocytic anemias, e.g. suspicion of intravascular hemolysis, blood loss,
- monitoring the response to therapy in deficiency anemias, e.g. iron, vitamin C, vitamin B_6, vitamin B_{12}, folate deficiency,
- evaluation of erythropoiesis after erythropoietin therapy.

The reticulocyte count is expressed either as a percentage (number of reticulocytes/1000 red cells) or as an absolute cell count (reticulocytes/µl).

Reference interval reticulocyte count [132]:

Relative proportion	
• Children and adults	5-15‰
Absolute (10^3/µl)	
• Adults	30--100

Daily RBC replacement (40,000 to 50,000/µl) represents 0.5 to 1.5 % of the total RBC count. These cells can be identified as polychromatophilic cells on routine staining (e.g., Wright's or Giemsa stain colors remnants of RNA) or as reticulocytes on supravital staining, which recognizes endoplasmic reticular material within the cells. The reticulocyte count is done by taking a few drops of blood initially stained with fresh methylene blue, then counterstained with Wright's stain. Under oil immersion, the numbers of 1000 consecutive RBCs having a blue-staining reticulum are counted and expressed as a percentage (normally 0.5 to 1.5 %). Reticulocytes may be enumerated using automated differential counters.

Because reticulocytes represent a young cell population, the reticulocyte count is an important criterion of marrow activity that can be considered a response to a need for RBC renewal. An increased reticulocyte count (reticulocytosis) suggests a restoration response after acute blood loss or specific therapy for anemias caused by deficient erythropoiesis (i.e., vitamin B_{12}, folic acid, and iron-deficiency anemias). Reticulocytosis is particularly prominent in hemolytic anemias and in acute and severe bleeding. A normal reticulocyte count in anemia indicates failure of the bone marrow to respond appropriately. Such a reticulocytopenia is usually caused by a nutrient or hormonal deficiency resulting in deficient erythropoiesis; one dramatic mechanism is the presence of viral infections (especially human parvovirus B19) as a cause for severe, but transient, decreased RBC production.

Reticulocyte Maturity Index (RMI)

The RMI in peripheral blood depends on the extent of the anemia, the status of the illness and the iron status.

The RMI which is independent from the reticulocyte count serves as an indicator of the erythropoietic bone marrow activity and allows anemias to be further sub-classified.

Tests for the Diagnosis of Disorders of Iron Metabolism

In addition to hematological the following laboratory tests are also indispensable in the differential diagnosis of disturbances of iron metabolism.

The following parameters are available in routine laboratory testing:

- Hemoglobin (Hb)
- Iron
- Total iron-binding capacity (TIBC)
  Latent iron-binding capacity (LIBC)
- Ferritin
- Transferrin (Tf)
  Transferrin saturation (TfS)
- Soluble Transferrin receptor (s-TfR)
- Zinc protoporphyrin
- Haptoglobin (Hp)
- Ceruloplasmin (Cp)
- Folic acid / vitamin B12
- Erythropoietin (EPO)

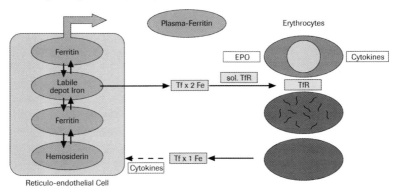

Fig. 43. Iron metabolism
According to Sunder-Plassmann and W. H. Hörl Clin. Lab. 1996; 42: 269-277

Table 35. Concentration ranges of the analysis

Parameter	Reference concentration intervals		Analytical method
	[μg/dl]	[μmol/l]	
Iron	40-160	7-29*	Spectrophotometry
Iron-binding capacity (TIBC)	260-500	46-90	Spectrophotometry
Transferrin	200 000-400 000 (= 2-4 g/l)	25-50**	Immunochemical method
Soluble transferrin receptor (s-TfR)	500-3000 (= 0.5-3 mg/l)	$6\text{-}35 \times 10^{-3}$***	Immunochemical method
Ferritin	1-30 (= 10-300 ng/ml)	$0.2\text{-}7 \times 10^{-6}$****	Immunochemical method
Haptoglobin	60 000-270 000 (= 0.6-2.7 g/dl)	7-32*****	Immunochemical method
Ceruloplasmin (Cp)	15 000-60 000 (= 15-60 mg/dl)	$1,1\text{-}4,5$++++	Immunochemical method
Folic acid	0.2-2 (= 2.7-16.1 ng/ml)	$6\text{-}37 \times 10^{-3}$+	Immunochemical method
Vitamin B_{12}	$20\text{-}90 \times 10^{-3}$	$150\text{-}670 \times 10^{-6}$++	Immunochemical method
Erythropoietin (EPO)	6-25 IU/l		Immunochemical method

	Rel. mol. weight of hemoglobin:	68,000 daltons
*	Rel. atomic weight of iron:	56 daltons
**	Rel. mol. weight of transferrin:	79,570 daltons (apotransferrin)
***	Rel. mol. weight of transferrin receptor:	85,000 daltons
****	Rel. mol. weight of ferritin:	440,000 daltons
*****	Rel. mol. weight of haptoglobin:	100,000 daltons Hp 1-1
		200,000 daltons Hp 2-1
		400,000 daltons Hp 2-2
+	Rel. mol. weight of folic acid:	445 daltons
++	Rel. mol. weight of vitamin B_{12}:	1355 daltons
+++	Rel. mol. weight of erythropoietin:	34,000 daltons
++++	Rel. mol. weight of ceruloplasmin:	132,000 daltons

Free iron ions do not occur in the blood. The so-called plasma or serum iron is almost entirely transferrin-bound. Because of its technical simplicity, the determination of transferrin has displaced the determination of the iron-binding capacity. Ferritin is the depot protein, which occurs not only intracellularly, but also (in very low concentrations) in the blood.

In macrocytic anemias the simultaneous determination of folic acid and vitamin B_{12} is nowadays a routine method of laboratory diagnosis.

Determination of Iron

In addition to the colorimetric methods, which are by far the most commonly used, atomic absorption spectrophotometry (AAS) and potentiostatic coulometry are also available as special techniques. More than 90% of all iron determinations in clinical laboratories are performed colorimetrically, in most cases using routine analyzers.

All the colorimetric methods developed for the determination of iron have the following steps in common:

– *Liberation* of the Fe^{3+} ions from the transferrin complex by acids or tensides.

In some methods, the liberation of Fe^{3+} ions by acid is combined with deproteinization after addition of trichloroacetic acid or chloroform. Deproteinization is unnecessary if a suitable tenside (e.g., guanidinium chloride) is used in a weakly acidic solution (pH 5). The liberation of Fe^{3+} by a tenside *without* deproteinization has the advantages that there is no turbidity due to incomplete deproteinization, the removal of Fe^{3+} from the transferrin is complete, and hemoglobin-bound Fe^{2+} is not liberated.

– *Reduction* of Fe^{3+} ions to Fe^{2+} ions

To enable the color reaction with a suitable chromophore to take place, the Fe^{3+} ions must first be reduced. Ascorbate has proved to be a particularly suitable reducing agent; hydroquinone, thioglycolate, and hydroxylamine are also used.

– *Reaction* of the Fe^{2+} ions to form a color complex

The only complexing agents used nowadays are bathophen-anthroline and Ferro Zine (registered trade name, Hach Chemical Co., Ames, Iowa/USA). Ferro Zine has a higher extinction coefficient than bathophenanthroline and its solubility is also better. Slightly higher iron values are obtained with Ferro Zine.

Methods

At present there is no reference method for the determination of serum/plasma iron. However, reference methods have been proposed by the International Committee for Standardization in Hematology (ICSH) [60, 61] and more recently by the Center of Disease Control (CDC).

The method recommended by the ICSH uses 2 mol/l hydrochloric acid for the liberation of the Fe^{3+} ions and thioglycolic acid for the reduction. The complexing agent is bathophenanthroline-disulphonate.

Table 36. Historical survey

Year	Milestone
1958	Bathophenanthroline method without deproteinization (Sanford und Ramsay)
1972	Bathophenanthroline method (ICSH recommendation)
1990	Ferro Zine method *with* deproteinization (CDC recommendation)
1998	Ferro Zine method *without* deproteinization

The CDC proposal is a method *with* deproteinization by trichloroacetic acid, and with reduction by ascorbic acid. The complexing agent is Ferro Zine.

In the Ferro Zine method *without* deproteinization, the reaction is measured in the cuvette itself. The Ferro Zine iron complex formed can be measured in the wavelength range from 530 to 560 nm by any routine analyzer.

Sample Material

Every serum sample contains the five iron fractions listed in Table 37.

Table 37. Iron fractions

Fractions	Iron concentration in serum	
*Tri*valent iron in transferrin	$\approx$ 50-150 µg/dl	Fe^{3+}
*Di*valent iron in hemoglobin	5-10 µg/dl	Fe^{2+}
*Tri*valent iron in ferritin	0.2-10 µg/dl	Fe^{3+}
Complexed iron	< 0.5 µg/dl	Fe^{2+}/Fe^{3+}
Iron ions due to contamination	<< 0.5 µg/dl	Fe^{3+}/Fe^{2+}

The iron level shows a distinct circadian rhythm. There is also a considerable day-to-day variation. Serum iron is protein-bound. The collection of blood samples must therefore be standardized with respect to time, body position and venous occlusion. Iron is one of the trace elements, with a concentration similar to those of copper and zinc. Contamination must therefore be avoided during the collection and preparation of samples (Fig. 42).

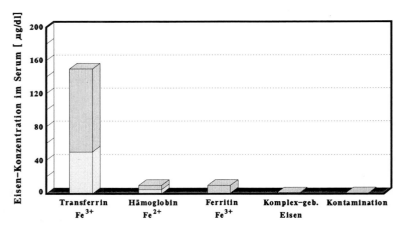

Fig. 44. Distribution of plasma iron

Serum and heparinized plasma are suitable for use as samples. EDTA plasma cannot be used. Hemolysis interferes. No detectable change in the iron concentration is found upon storage of serum for several weeks at +4°C.

Reference range for serum/plasma iron [51]:

Women	37-145 [μg/dl]	6.6-26 [μmol/l]
Men	59-158 [μg/dl]	11-28 [μmol/l]

Notes on Iron Reference Range

Considerable differences are found in the reference ranges given in the literature for iron. There are various reasons for this:
– The reference range does not have a normal distribution.
– The iron level decreases significantly with increasing age.
– Iron concentrations found for men are about 15 to 20% higher than those for women.
– Iron concentrations are high in babies, but decrease from the 2nd to the 3rd year of life.

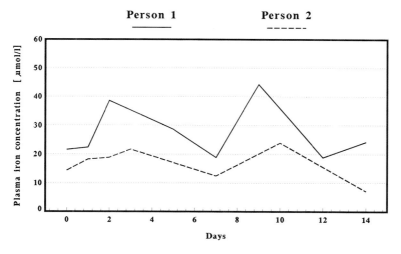

Fig. 45. Day to day fluctuations of the plasma iron concentration

–   The plasma iron level has a pronounced circadian rhythm.
    The difference between morning and evening values can be
up to 50 µg/dl. Day-to-day and week-to-week variations in
    the same individual are also very pronounced.

Iron Saturation
= Total Iron-Binding Capacity (TIBC) and the
Latent Iron-Binding Capacity (LIBC)

These methods have now been largely replaced by the determination of transferrin and of the transferrin saturation [44]. The
TIBC and the LIBC were used before the determination of
transferrin became technically easy to perform.

The TIBC is the quantity of iron that can be bound by transferrin in a specified volume of serum. This is an indirect way of
assessing transferrin levels.

The LIBC is the result obtained when the quantity of iron actually present is subtracted from the TIBC. It represents transferrin without iron.

The following relation exists:

TIBC = LIBC + plasma iron

The TIBC is measured in the routine laboratory according to
Ramsay, and is performed in parallel with the determination of
iron.

An excess of Fe^{3+} ions is added to the serum to saturate the
transferrin. The unbound Fe^{3+} ions are then precipitated with basic magnesium carbonate. After centrifugation, the iron in the
clear supernatant is measured.

Determination of Iron-Binding Proteins: Immunoassay Methods

The modern methods for the determination of Plasma proteins are based on immunoassays. The principle is still relatively new, but its importance is rapidly growing, and a brief description will therefore be given [82].

Immunoassay Methods

All methods for the determination of plasma proteins such as ferritin and transferrin are based on the immunological principle of the reaction between an antigen (AG) and an antibody (AB). Following the addition of a suitable antiserum, this reaction leads to the formation of an immune complex of the antigen (the protein to be determined) and the antibody:

$$AG + AB = AGAB$$
$$AG = antigen, AB = antibody$$

In immunological methods, antibodies are used as reagents for the determination of the analyte. The antibodies used must have a high specificity as well as high affinity for the antigen.

A distinction is made between *polyclonal* antibodies, which are mixtures from different cell lines, and *monoclonal* antibodies, which are derived from a single cell line. The latter are produced by the procedure published by Köhler and Milstein, and are

Table 38. Indirect measurement of the primary immuno-reaction after labeling

	Assay
Enzymes	Enzyme immunoassay (EIA)
Radioactive isotope	Radioimmunoassay (RIA)
Fluorescent dye	Fluorescence immunoassay (FIA)
Luminescence-producing substances	Luminescence immunoassay (LIA)

Table 39. Direct measurement methods

	Assay
Measurement of the precipitate in solution	Turbidimetric immunoassay
	Nephelometric immunoassay
Measurement of the agglutination of coated particles	Latex immunoagglutination assays
Precipitate in gels	Radial immunodiffusion

identical in their antigen specificity and in their antigen-binding behavior [75].

The initially formed antigen-antibody complex cannot be observed directly if the antigen concentration is very low. In this case either the antigen or the antibody must be labeled in order to make a measurement possible. The label may be e.g. an enzyme, a radioactive isotope, or a fluorescent dye. These indirect methods are particularly suitable for the determination of very low antigen concentrations, as in the case of ferritin.

With higher antigen concentrations, the initial reaction between the antigen and the antibody may be followed by agglutination or precipitation as a secondary reaction. The results can then be measured directly, and are often visible. The direct methods are particularly suitable for determination of higher antigen concentrations, as e.g. in the case of transferrin.

The immunochemical methods used for the determination of analytes in routine laboratory work can be divided into indirect methods with labeling and direct methods [82]. The use of labels enables the automated measurement of the primary immunoreaction.

The radioimmunoassay was introduced in 1956 by Berson and Yalow. Enzyme immunoassays, fluorescence immunoassays [82], and luminescence immunoassays followed later as logical developments designed to avoid the disadvantages associated with the use of radioactive materials. The quantitative determination of all direct immunoassays is based on the Heidelberger-Kendall curve [50], which describes the relationship between the

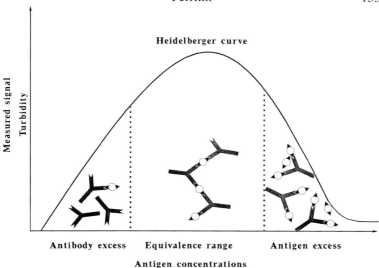

Fig. 46. Heidelberger-Kendall curve: Relationship between
quantity of antigen and measured signal or quantity of precipitate

antigen concentration and the quantity of precipitate for a constant quantity of antibody. The quantity of precipitate is measured (Fig. 43).

The ratio of the antigen concentration to the antibody concentration is particularly important in the direct methods, since this ratio directly influences the formation of the precipitate.

As can be seen from the course of the Heidelberger curve, two different antigen concentrations can give the same measurement signal. This can lead to incorrect results. Quantitative immunoassays must therefore be performed below the equivalence point. The conventional method of deciding whether a signal lies on the ascending (antibody excess) or descending (antigen excess) part of the Heidelberger curve is to repeat the determination with a higher dilution of the sample. Another possibility is to add antigen or antiserum to the reaction mixture. Modern automated analyzers can virtually eliminate this source of error by means of check functions (characterization and au-

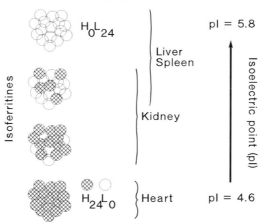

Fig. 47. Organ-specific isoferritins

tomatic redilution of the sample). Most manufacturers of immunochemical reagents declare the concentration range in which no antigen excess problem arises, i. e., no high-dose hook effect is found.

Ferritin

The ferritin that can be detected in the blood is in equilibrium with the body's storage iron, and can thus serve as an index [40, 69, 84] of the size of the iron stores.

Ferritin occurs in different tissues as various isoferritins. These isoferritins are constructed from two subunits, the H-(heavy)-type subunit and the L-(light)-type subunit (Fig. 44).

For the clinical evaluation of the body's iron stores by determination of the ferritin, the ferritin antibodies must possess specificity for the basic L-rich isoferritins from iron storage tissues (marrow, liver, spleen), whereas their reactivity with acidic H-rich isoferritins (e. g. from cardiac muscle) should be as low as possible.

Among the label-free immunoassay methods, latex-enhanced agglutination tests are particularly suitable for detection of the very low plasma ferritin concentration. Among the im-

Table 40. Historical survey

Year	Milestone
1972	Development of an immunoradiometric assay (IRMA), (Addison et al.)
1984	Turbidimetric test with reaction enhancement by latex (Bernard et al.)
1984	ICSH ferritin standard defined
1997	3rd International Standard for Ferritin, NIBSC code 95/572 (Thorpe et al.)

munoassay methods with labels, enzyme immunoassays (EIAs), FIAs, and RIAs are widely used.

Ferritin in plasma/serum must be determined in a very low concentration range ($0.2\text{-}10 \times 10^{12}$ mol/l). A sufficiently sensitive method is therefore essential. The list of milestones for ferritin shows that the first generation of tests were all based on an indirect measurement of the primary immune reaction using labels (radioimmunoassay, enzyme immunoassay). In recent years, the sensitivity of the direct methods (turbidimetry, nephelometry) has been improved considerably [82].

Parallel to the development of the methods, success was also achieved in efforts to automate the various direct and indirect immunochemical methods.

There is (at present) no reference method for the determination of ferritin.

International efforts towards a uniform standardization of ferritin are being coordinated by the WHO (World Health Organization), the ICSH (International Committee of Standardization in Hematology), the IFCC (International Federation of Clinical Chemistry), and the IUIS (Standardization Committee of the International Union of Immunological Societies).

The prerequisite for uniform standardization is a defined ferritin preparation with a high content of basic isoferritins. The ICHS (Expert Panel of Iron) has had a defined ferritin standard (human liver ferritin) since 1984. Since 1997 the WHO 3rd

Table 41. Ferritin methods

Method
Turbidimetric latex agglutination test
Enzyme-linked immunosorbent assay (ELISA)
Nephelometric immunoassay
Fluorescence immunoassay (FIA)
Luminescence immunoassay (LIA)
Radioimmunoassay (RIA)

International Standard for Ferritin, recombinant (94/572) has been available [135].

In view of the vast number of commercially available methods, a decision in favor of a given method can only be reached after consideration of several criteria, depending on the size of the laboratory:

Types and numbers of samples,

Urgency of the request (STAT), speed of the determination

Specificity, sensitivity, precision,

Possibility of automation, personnel required, cost per determination

Many of the modern commercially available ferritin methods exhibit good specificity, precision, and sensitivity within their field of application and show good agreement in comparisons with one another (Fig. 45).

A homogeneous immunoassay can be performed with the existing Integra-or Hitachi-routine analyzers. Intelligent, user-friendly automation of Heterogenes Immunological (Cobas Core or Elecsys) has been developed.

Ferritin, like transferrin, but unlike iron, shows no appreciable circadian rhythm. In view of the effect of an upright body position on high molecular weight blood components, the blood collection conditions must be standardized with regard to body position and venous occlusion.

Preferably the same sample should be used for the ferritin determinations as for the iron and transferrin.

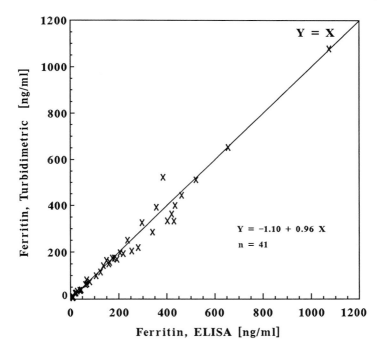

Fig. 48. Comparison of turbidimetric and elecsys methods for the determination of ferritin

Reference Range

The determination of reference ranges for the ferritin concentrations of clinically healthy individuals is extremely difficult [30], since iron stores are strongly dependent on age and sex (Fig. 46), and a significant fraction of the „normal population" suffers from *latent* iron deficiency. This limits the usefulness of selected reference groups, such as regular blood donors, or individuals subject to military service, or even young female

Ferritin concentrations in healthy individuals

Men	30 - 400 ng/ml	$0.7 - 10 \times 10^{-6}$ µmol/l
Women under 50 years of age	15 - 150 ng/ml	$0.3 - 4 \times 10^{-6}$ µmol/l
Women over 50 years of age	Approximation to the reference interval for men	

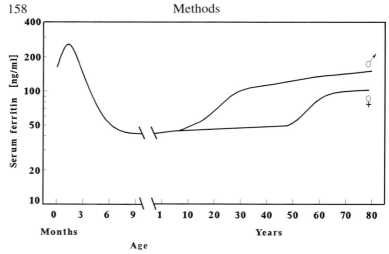

Fig. 49. Age and sex dependence of the serum ferritin concentration[Dallmann et al. (1980) Am J Clin Nutr 33:86]

hospital staff. The reference values listed have been compiled from several studies with well-defined „normal study populations". In particular, individuals with iron deficiency anemia (manifest iron deficiency) and infections (clinical examination, laboratory results) were excluded.

Babies initially have full iron stores, which are used up within a few weeks.
The indicated reference ranges statistically cover 95% of clinically healthy population groups. They do not by any means represent an ideal norm, and are not suitable for use as decision criteria related to therapy.

Transferrin (Tf)

Half of the body's transferrin is contained in the serum/plasma, while the other half is extravascular. The protein is able to transport two trivalent iron ions per molecule. 30 to 40% of this maximum binding capacity is utilized under physiological conditions.

Table 42. Historical survey

Year	Milestones
1958	Determination of transferrin by radial immunodiffusion, RID
1965	Quantitative determination by RID
1976	Turbidimetric determination of transferrin (Kreutzer)
1978	Nephelometric determination (Buffone et al.)

Transferrin is a group of various isotransferrins. Presently approximately 20 human isotransferrins are known. They all have the same iron-binding capacity and similar immunological characteristics. Therefore distinguishing between the various isoforms has no practical value for the assessment of iron metabolism. Since the technical requirements for the determination of transferrin in the routine laboratory are relatively simple, the determination of the tansferrin in serum/plasma has displaced the determination of the TIBC (total iron-binding capacity) and of the LIBC (latent iron-binding capacity).

Transferrin, like ferritin, but unlike iron, shows no pronounced circadian rhythm. In view of the effect of an upright body position on high molecular weight blood components, the blood collection conditions for transferrin determinations must again be standardized with regard to body position and vein constriction.

Preferably the same sample should be used for the transferrin determination as for iron and ferritin.

Reference range for transferrin [51]:

Transferrin concentration	2.0-4.0 [g/l]	25-50 [μmol/l]
in healthy individuals	200-400 [mg/dl]	

No great dependence on age or sex is found.

Relationship between Transferrin and Total Iron Binding Capacity (TIBC)

Table 43. Relationship between transferrin and TIBC [44]

Relationship between transferrin and TIBC	Reference ranges [51]
Transferrin [µmol/l] x 2 ~ TIBC [µmol/l]	Transferrin: 25-50 [µmol/l] w; TIBC; 49-89 [µmol/l] m: TIBC: 52-77 [µmol/l]
Transferrin [µg/dl] x $\frac{2x56}{79570}$ ~ TIBC [µg/dl]	Transferrin: 200-400 [mg/dl] w; TIBC; 274-497 [µg/dl] m: TIBC: 291-430 [µg/dl]
Transferrin [mg/dl] x 1.41 ~ TIBC [µg/dl]	TIBC: 300-600 [µg/dl]

The following has been taken into account:
1 mol of transferrin binds 2 atoms of iron
Atomic weight of iron = 56 daltons
Molecular weight of APO transferrin = 79,570 daltons [48]
Remark: Total Iron Binding Capacity (TIBC) of 1 g transferrin is 1.41 mg iron.

Transferrin Saturation (TfS)

Transferrin saturation is defined as the ratio of the serum/plasma iron concentration to the serum/plasma transferrin concentration (multiplied by a correction factor)[44]. It is a dimensionless quantity, so that unlike iron, it is independent of the patient's state of hydration:

Transferrin saturation in % $\quad = \quad \dfrac{\text{Iron } [\mu\text{mol/l}] \times 100}{\text{Transferrin } [\mu\text{mol/l}]}$

or:

Transferrin saturation in % $\quad = \quad \dfrac{\text{Iron } [\mu\text{g/dl}] \times 100 \times 56}{\text{Transferrin } [\mu\text{g/dl}] \times 79570}$

$$\dfrac{\text{Iron } [\mu\text{g/dl}] \times 100 \times 56 \times 1000}{\text{Transferrin } [\text{mg/dl}] \times 79570}$$

$$\dfrac{\text{Iron } [\mu\text{g/dl}] \times 100}{\text{Transferrin } [\text{mg/dl}] \times 1{,}41}$$

Remarks

56	Atomic weight of iron in daltons
79 570	Molecular weight of APO transferrin in daltons

Reference range for transferrin saturation: [51]

Transferrin saturation in healthy individuals	15-45 %
Decreased transferrin saturation in iron deficiency or disturbances of iron distribution	< 15 %
Elevated transferrin saturation in iron overload	> 45 %

Remarks

Transferrin saturation of 10 % expresses that 1 g transferrin is saturated with 0.141 mg Iron.

Transferrin saturation of 50 % is reached, when 1 g transferrin contains 0.705 mg iron.

Methods

There is (at present) no reference method for the determination of transferrin.

Because of the relatively high transferrin concentration (25-50 μmol/l), direct immunological precipitation methods (neph-elometry, turbidimetry] are suitable. Turbidimetric and nephelo-metric methods are widely used as routine methods. It is difficult to make any general recommendation for one particular test, in view of the many commercial methods available.

Transferrin Receptor (TfR)

For transportation of iron in plasma the Fe^{3+}-protein complex now binds to a specific transferrin receptor, which is located on the cell surface, and to then internalized by endocytosis.

In all cell types Fe^{3+} import is regulated via the expression of that receptor. However, 80 % of the transferrin receptors are found on the surface of erythroid marrow. The receptor is a dimer with a molecular weight of about 190 kDa, whose each subunit is able to bind one molecule of transferrin.

A smaller part of the transferrin receptors – the soluble transferrin receptors (sTfR) are found in the plasma. The sTfR is a truncated form of the tissue receptor with a molecular weight of 85 kDa.

It is suggested that the soluble form is produced by proteolytic cleavage of the two extracellular arms of the intact transmembrane receptor [20, 21, 59].

Although a lot of groups are working on that field, the biological function of sTfR is not yet completely understood.

However, it was found out that the concentration of the sTfR is directly correlated to the concentration of the cell surface-bound receptor molecules. So its concentration provides us with an excellent tool for the measurement of the erythroid precursor mass and gives us information about the real severity of tissue iron deficiency.

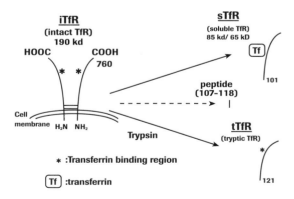

Fig. 50. Schematic presentation of soluble
Transferrin receptor (s-TfR)

The soluble serum transferrin receptor released into the blood is a monomer of approximately 85,000 daltons. It is produced after the proteolytic splitting of approximately 100 amino acids to N-terminus [21, 59].

The diagnosis of iron deficiency is relatively straight forward in patients who are otherwise fit and can be made after determining such parameters as ferritin, total iron binding capacity and serum iron to assess the patient's iron status. The diagnosis is more complicated in patients with chronic disease because chronic diseases have a direct influence on ion status markers. Chronic disease can in particular lead to the detection of normal serum ferritin values in patients suffering from iron deficiency whereas in patients with sufficient reserves of iron, serum iron values are depressed. It has been shown that in this group of patients the soluble transferrin receptor in serum (sTfR) is of comparable diagnostic value to a bone marrow aspirate in identifying iron deficient patients. The concept is based on two facts: expression of transferrin receptors is proportional to the cellular iron demand, i.e. it is elevated in iron deficiency and the sTfR serum level is proportional to the total amount of cellular transferrin receptors [20, 21, 106, 107].

The exact determination of the iron status is extremely important because iron deficiency is often the main symptom of gastrointestinal bleeding which may be due to a non-diagnosed malignant tumor. Timely differentiation between iron deficiency anemia and anemia of chronic disease can under certain circumstances lead to the saving of life because patients with anemia

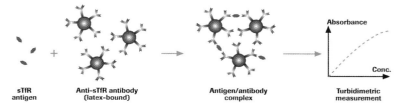

Fig. 51. Test principle of Particle-enhanced immunoturbidimetric assay of soluble Transferrin receptor (s-TfR)

during chronic disease can be identified correctly and further tests can be performed. When evaluating the iron status of patients with concomitant chronic disease, the soluble transferrin receptor test should be performed.

Methods

There is still no reference method for determining the soluble serum transferrin receptor.

On account of the relatively low concentration of soluble serum transferrin receptor in the blood (< 10 mg/l or < 100 nmol/l), only sufficiently sensitive measuring methods are suitable for the determination.

Latex-enhanced turbidimetric homogeneous immunoassay for the quantitative in vitro determination of the soluble transferrin receptor in human sera and plasma are the method most frequently used for routine determinations.

The sTfR-molecule from the sample reacts with the latex particles coated with anti-sTfR-antibodies (monoclonal, mouse) and forms an antigen/antibody complex which is then measured turbidimetrically.

As sample material serum and plasma can be used. No sample preparation is necessary. Following anticoagulatns are accepted: Li-heparin, Na-heparin, no EDTA plasma and citrate plasma can be used.

Preliminary Reference Range

In a study a collective of 96 patients (58 men and 38 women) have been tested. All patients had been checked before for normal kidney function (by determining creatinine), for normal ferritin concentration (determined by transferrin saturation), and of exclusion of an acute phase reaction (by determining CRP). The 2.5 % and 97.5 % percentile has been calculated then of the remaining 96 patients [76].

The study resulted in a preliminary normal range of:

2.16 – 4.54 mg/L, n = 58

and for women 1.79 – 4.63 mg/L, n = 38

Table 44. Historical survey

Year	Milestones
1960	Haptoglobin-hemoglobin binding test; determination of free haptoglobin in serum (Nyman)
1965	Radial immunodiffusion RID (Fahey et al.)
1979	Nephelometric determination of haptoglobin
1987	Turbidimetric test for haptoglobin (Johnson)

Haptoglobin

The haptoglobin detectable in the serum binds the hemoglobin resulting from pathologically increased hemolysis in a fixed haptoglobin-hemoglobin (Hp-Hb) complex. A decrease in the free haptoglobin thus serves as an indicator of intravascular hemolysis.

The 1:1 Hp-Hb complex is incorporated into the hepatocytes with a half-life of less than 10 min. There, the hemoglobin is enzymatically metabolized. The haptoglobin released is returned to the serum with a half-life of about 3 days.

The formation of the fixed Hp-Hb complex and its extremely rapid elimination from the bloodstream prevents hemoglobinuria with severe renal iron loss.

Haptoglobin is a glycoprotein structurally related to the immunoglobulins, and is made up of 2 light (α-)chains with a molecular weight of 9000 daltons and two heavier (β-)chains (molecular weight: 16,000 daltons). Three phenotypes with different molecular weights are known: Hp 1-1, Hp 2-1 and Hp 2-2. Hp 1-1 has a molecular weight of 100,000 daltons. Hp 2-1 and Hp 22 are high-molecular-weight polymers with a molecular weight ranging from 200,000 to 400,000 daltons.

There is (at present) no reference method for the determination of haptoglobin. Because of the relatively high haptoglobin concentration in the serum (7-32 µmol/l), direct immunological precipitation methods (e.g., radial immunodiffusion, nephelometry, turbidimetry) are suitable. Turbidimetric and nephelometric methods are widely used as routine methods [95].

Reference range for haptoglobin* [51]:

Adults	30-200 [mg/dl]	0.3-2.0 [g/l]

*CRM 470 standardized

Haptoglobin concentrations in the serum of healthy persons. There are no major differences based on age or sex.

Remarks:
Neonates have no measurable haptoglobin levels in the first 3 months; the reference range for adults applies from the 4th month. The reference range is dependent on the phenotype:

	[g/l]	[mg/dl]
Hp 1-1	0.7-2.3	70-230
Hp 2-1	0.9-3.6	90-360
Hp 2-2	0.6-2.9	60-290

Like the ferritin and transferrin level, that of haptoglobin shows no appreciable circadian rhythm. In view of the effect of an upright body position on high molecular weight blood components, the blood collection conditions must be standardized with regard to body position and venous occlusion. The haptoglobin determination should preferably be performed using the same serum sample as for the other iron metabolism parameters.

In presence of massive hemolysis – when no haptoglobin concentration is detectable - hemopexin (Hpx) should be measured [95].

Ceruloplasmin (Cp)

Cp is a glycoprotein with a molecular mass of 132 kDa and contains about 9% carbohydrate. The Cp molecule binds 6-8 Cu atoms.

Cp is an α_2-glycoprotein which is synthesized mostly in the liver. Its functions include:
- transport of copper (Cu) in plasma
- ferroxidase activity; it oxidizes Fe^{2+} to Fe^{3+}
- antioxidative effect, due to the prevention of metal ion-catalyzed oxidation of lipids in the cell membrane
- acute phase protein in inflammation.

Methods of determination for routine use are: immunonephelometry and immunoturbidimetry.

Reference range for ceruloplasmin* [51]:

Adults	15-60 mg/dl or 0,15-0,6g/l

*CRM 470 standardized

The most important physiological functions of Cp are:
- regulation of transport, availability, and redox potential of iron (Fe) as a result of its ferroxidase activity. For instance, if functional iron is required for erythropoiesis, Fe^{3+} is released from ferritin via reduction to Fe^{2+}. However, since the transport protein transferrin can only bind Fe^{3+}, Fe^{2+} is immediately oxidized to Fe^{3+} by Cp.
- prevention of metal-ion-catalyzed peroxidation of membrane lipids. This peroxidation is thought to be a causative cofactor of many disorders such as atherosclerosis or neurotoxicity. Cp reacts either directly with the superoxide anions or oxidizes Fe^{2+} or Cu^{2+} and thus prevents peroxidation of lipids.
- specific transport of copper

New insights have been gained concerning the role of ceruloplasmin in iron metabolism. This copper transporting protein seems to be important for intracellular oxidation of Fe^{2+} to Fe^{3+} which is necessary for release of iron ions from the cells and the binding to transferrin. This is exemplified by the very rare hereditary aceruloplasminemia where the lack of iron oxidation prevents binding to transferrin and thereby leads to intracellular trapping of iron ions and consequently to the development of an iron overload which resembles hereditary hemochromatosis. However, in contrast to hemochromatosis the central nervous system is also affected. Due to the impaired transferrin binding, however, iron concentrations and transferrin saturation in plasma are low whereas ferritin concentrations are high, reflecting the impaired iron distribution and release.

Determination of Vitamin B12 and Folic Acid

The diagnostic value of determining vitamin B_{12} and folic acid in anemic states -in addition to serum ferritin- is increasingly appreciated, and is beyond dispute. All modern vitamin B_{12} and folate determinations in serum are based on an immunological analysis method.

Because the indication is the same in virtually all cases, it is customary and often useful to determine folic acid and vitamin B_{12} in the plasma simultaneously as a double assay.

Vitamin B12

Vitamin B_{12} has a molecular weight of 1355 daltons and, as cyanocobalamin, belongs to a biologically active substance group which has as common structural element a porphyrin ring with cobalt as the central atom.

The vitamin B12 taken in with food or synthesized by intestinal bacteria („extrinsic factor") forms a complex with the „intrinsic factor", a glycoprotein formed in the gastric mucosa. Formation of this complex serves to protect the vitamin from degradation in the intestine and facilitates its receptor-dependent absorption by the mucosa of the small intestine. After dissociation of the vitamin B12 „intrinsic-factor" complex the vitamin can be transported to the liver, where it is stored. In the cells the vitamin is present mainly as 5'deoxyadenosyl-cobalamin, whereas methylcobalamin predominates in the plasma. Transcobalamin II (TC-II) serves as the most important transport protein for vitamin B12 in the plasma.

Table 45. Historical survey

Year	Milestones
1950	Microbiological determination of Lactobacillus Leichmannii (Mathews)
1961	Radioimmunological determination (Bavakat, Ekins)
1978	Use of highly purified intrinsic factor as binding protein (Kolhouse et al.)
1986	Automated determination of B_{12}/folate (Henderson et al.)

A microbiological assay is recommended by the NCCLS as reference method for the research laboratory. The biological activity of vitamin B_{12} is measured in relation to the growth of the microorganisms E. gracilis or L. Leichmannii. It is not suitable for wider use because of the apparatus required and the specificity of the technique.

A considerable advance in methods was made in 1962 with the introduction of a radioimmunoassay. The determination is based on the competitive binding of radiolabeled vitamin B_{12} and the free vitamin B_{12} in the sample to the intrinsic factor. Before the determination is performed, vitamin B_{12} is released from the endogenous binding proteins in a thermal stage or by pretreatment in an alkaline solution.

The method described by Kolhouse et al. in 1978 makes it possible to exclude binding of endogenous cobalamin analogs in the serum to nonspecific R proteins in the immunological test.

Serum/plasma vitamin B_{12} must be determined in a very low concentration range (50-1500 pg/ml). This calls for a sufficiently sensitive method. The list of milestones shows that the first generation of determination methods was based exclusively on indirect measurement by radioimmunoassay. In 1986 Henderson, Friedman et al. introduced a non-radioactive immunoassay.

Reference range for vitamin B_{12} [51]:

Adults	220-925 pg/ml	(162-683 pmol/l)

Vitamin B_{12} concentrations in the serum of healthy persons. There are no major differences based on age or sex.
Remarks:
In about 20% of pregnant women, the vitamin B_{12} concentration in the serum falls to values of < 125 pmol/l despite adequate depots.

Some of the reference ranges for vitamin B_{12} given in the literature differ considerably. This is undoubtedly due to the considerable differences in methods used in the past.

Table 46. Historical survey

Year	Milestones
1966	Microbiological determination of N-5-methyl-tetrahydrofolic acid (MTHFA) with Lactobacillus casei (Herbert)
1973	Determination of folic acid by radioimmunoassay (Dunn et al., Rothenberg et al.)
1977	Simultaneous determination of folate/B$_{12}$ (Gutcho, Mansbach)

Folic Acid

Folic acid is a pteridine derivative and is present as a conjugate with several glutaminic acid molecules (n = 2-7). After the ingestion of food it is initially hydrolyzed enzymatically to pteroylmonoglutaminic acid (PGA, molecular weight 441 daltons) in the mucosal epithelium of the small intestine. Reduction and methylation then take place in the intestinal wall; the resultant N-5-methyl-tetrahydrofolic acid (MTHFA, molecular weight 459 daltons) is released into the bloodstream. Tetrahydrofolic acid (THFA, molecular weight 445 daltons) is formed from METHFA under the influence of vitamin B$_{12}$. It is involved in numerous reactions as a coenzyme.

The microbiological assay recommended as reference method is unsuitable for widespread use. Measurements are made of the biological activity of N-5-methyltetrahydrofolic acid (MTHFA) in relation to the growth of Lactobacillus casei. An HPLC method developed by Gregory in 1985 is not suitable for the quantitative determination of folic acid in the serum, since it is not sufficiently sensitive.

A major advance in methods was achieved in 1973 with the introduction of the radioimmunological competitive protein binding test. The determination is based on the competitive binding of radiolabeled N-5-methyltetrahydrofolic acid (MTH-FA) (^{125}I-MTHFA) and the N-5-methyltetrahydrofolic acid (MTHFA) of the sample to the binding protein β-lactoglobulin. Before the determination is performed, MTHFA is released from the endogenous binding proteins in a thermal stage or by pretreatment in an alkaline solution. The false normal

results observed in individual cases which, compared with the microbiological reference method, failed to reveal a folic acid deficiency, can be corrected by using a chromatographically highly purified β-lactoglobulin free from nonspecific binding proteins.
Serum/plasma folic acid must be determined in a very low concentration range (0.5-20 ng/ml). This calls for a sufficiently sensitive method. The list of milestones shows that the first generation of determination methods was based exclusively on indirect measurement with a radioimmunoassay.Immunoassays have recently become commercially available which do not use radioisotopes but employ an elegant, simple reaction for separating folic acid from the endogenous binding proteins.

Reference range for folic acid [51]:

Adults	2,7-16,1 ng/ml	6,1-36,5 nmol/l)

There are no major differences based on age or sex.

Remarks:
Because of the close connection between vitamin B_{12} and folic acid in the metabolism and the difficulty of hematological and clinical differentiation between the two vitamin deficiency states, it is advisable to determine both parameters simultaneously in patients with the relevant vitamin deficiency symptoms.
The reference ranges for folic acid given in the literature differ considerably. This is undoubtedly due to the considerable differences in methods used in the past.

Erythropoietin (EPO)

Erythropoietin (EPO) is a glycoprotein with a molecular weight of 34,000 daltons. It contains a relatively high percentage of carbohydrates, at 60%.
EPO is a glycoprotein that controls a feedback mechanism to maintain a constant erythrocyte mass in the body. Increased

release of EPO leads to erythrocytosis and a reduction in erythrocytopenia.

In adults, 80-90% of EPO is formed in the kidneys.
Extrarenal formation sites include the liver and macrophages.
The kidney is merely a synthesis organ of EPO, i.e., it is synthe-
sized there as needed.

The focus of erythropoietin determination in clinical diagnostics lies in the differential diagnosis of erythrocytosis. The
significance of the differential diagnosis of anemias is increasing. Other indications are suspicion of renal anemia and determination of the starting value before initiating treatment of anemia with recombinant human EPO.

Methods

A reference method for the determination of erythropoietin
(EPO) does not exist at this time. Due to the extremely low concentration of EPO in serum, methods of determination must be
highly sensitive. Radio immunoassays and enzyme immunoassays which have been commercially available for about 5 years
are the most popular routine methods.

Sandwich Enzyme Immunoassay
The analytical sensitivity of the ELISA is 0.6 IU/l.

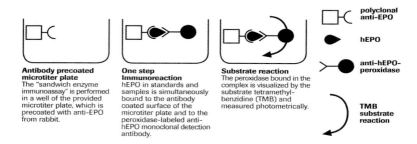

Antibody precoated microtiter plate
The "sandwich enzyme immunoassay" is performed in a well of the provided microtiter plate, which is precoated with anti-EPO from rabbit.

One step Immunoreaction
hEPO in standards and samples is simultaneously bound to the antibody coated surface of the microtiter plate and to the peroxidase-labeled anti-hEPO monoclonal detection antibody.

Substrate reaction
The peroxidase bound in the complex is visualized by the substrate tetramethyl-benzidine (TMB) and measured photometrically.

polyclonal anti-EPO

hEPO

anti-hEPO-peroxidase

TMB substrate reaction

Fig. 52. Test principle: Photometric enzyme immunoassay for the quantitative *in vitro* determination of human erythropoietin (EPO).

Interpretations of the measured EPO concentration is only possible in conjunction with hemoglobin or hematocrit levels. Interpretations of EPO reference ranges alone have no clinical relevance.

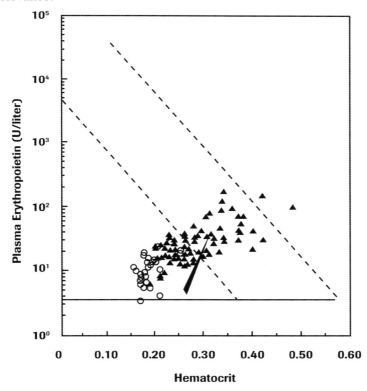

Fig. 53. Plasma erythropoietin levels in 120 patients receiving dialysis in relation to Hematocrit.
Open circles denote anephric patients and triangle patients with kidneys. The broken lines represent 95% confidence limits for 175 normal blood donors and patients with anemia. The solid line represents the limit of detection of the assay.
(From Ersley AJ: Erythropoietin. N Engl J Med 324: 1339-1344, 1991)

Reference range for Haptoglobin* [51]:

Adults	5-25 IU/l*

*related to the WHO 2nd International Reference Preparation for Bioassay (67/643)

Both a decrease and an increase in the production of EPO are of diagnostic significance. Both conditions can be detected by measuring serum EPO concentration.

EPO deficiency causes normocytic normochromic anemia. The most common cause is chronic renal failure because in adults EPO is almost exclusively synthesized in the kidney.

EPO overproduction occurs as a result of tissue hypoxia. In cases of non renal anemias, EPO concentration often increases exponentially as hemoglobin concentration decreases (Fig. 50).

Tests for the Diagnosis of Chronic Inflammation (ACD)

Laboratories are increasingly asked to differentiate between inflammatory and non-inflammatory diseases.

Inflammation can be detected using the following tests:
• Erythrocyte sedimentation rate (ESR)
• Quantitative determination of CRP and/or serum amyloid A protein (SAA)

The following tests are of additional relevance in the diagnosis of rheumatoid arthritis (RA):
• Determination of rheumatoid factor (RA)
• Iron/copper relation and ceruloplasmin
• Determination of other antibodies occurring in RA
  – Determination of antinuclear antibodies (ANA)
  – Determination of the antistreptolysin titer (ASL), and the antistreptococcus-desoxyribonuclease titer (ADNase)

In patients who fulfill the criteria for RA, the frequency of auto-antibodies in serum, particularly of antinuclear antibodies, varies. Detection of the above and other auto-antibodies should prompt further differential diagnostic considerations.

Erythrocyte Sedimentation Rate (ESR)

Method of Determination

A citrated blood sample is aspirated into a glass or plastic pipette with millimeter graduation up to the 200 mm mark. The pipette remains in an upright position and the sedimentation of red cells is read off in mm after one hour. The performance of the method follows an approved guideline.

Reference intervall [51]:

	Less than 50 years	More than 50 years
Women	< 25 mm/1 h	< 30 mm/1 h
Men	< 15 mm/1 h	< 20 mm/1 h

Values in mm for the first hour.*CRM 470 standardized

In comparison to the quantitative determination of an acute phase protein, e.g. CRP, the ESR is also raised by an increase in the concentration of immunoglobulins, immune complexes, and other proteins. It therefore covers a broader spectrum of diseases than CRP. In the case of chronic inflammatory disease, e.g. in SLE (systemic lupus erythematodes), in which CRP is often normal or only slightly elevated, and for monitoring in patients with these diseases, the ESR is therefore a better indicator of the inflammatory process.

C-Reactive Protein (CRP)

C-reactive protein is the classic acute phase protein that is released in response to an inflammatory reaction. It is synthesized in the liver.

CRP is composed of five identical, non-glycosylated subunits each comprising a single polypeptide chain of 206 amino acid residues with a molecular mass of 23,000 daltons. The characteristic structure places CRP in the family of pentraxins, calcium-binding proteins with immune defense properties.

CRP is synthesized rapidly in the liver following induction by IL-6. At the peak of an acute phase response, as much as 20% of the protein synthesizing capacity of the liver may be engaged in

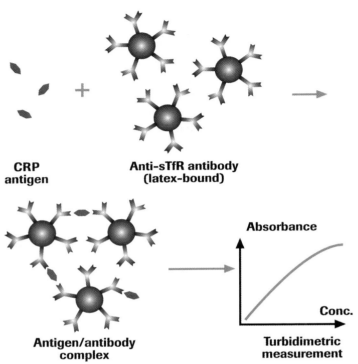

CRP antigen   **Anti-sTfR antibody (latex-bound)**

Antigen/antibody complex   **Turbidimetric measurement**

Fig. 54. Test principle of particle-enhanced immunoturbidimetric assay: Anti-CRP antibodies coupled to latex microparticles react with antigen in the sample to form an antigen/antibody complex. Following agglutination, this is measured turbidimetrically.

its synthesis. CRP levels increase in the plasma due to the release of inflammatory cytokines such as interleukin-6. Increased serum CRP levels are always an indicator of inflammation. However, malignancy such as M. Hodgkin, the kidney cell carcinoma, can also form these cytokines and prompt an acute phase response that induces fever and raised plasma concentrations of CRP.

CRP determination is used to screen for inflammatory processes:

- confirmation of the presence of acute organic disease such as infections, or chronic conditions or rheumatic diseases, and inflammatory bowel disease. For diagnosis and monitoring of infections when microbiological testing is too slow or impossible.
- As an indication of the presence of intercurrent infection in patients with some connective tissue diseases.
- As an aid in the management of rheumatic diseases.
- For rapid establishment of the optimal anti-inflammatory therapy and the determination of the minimal effective dose.

Methods of Determination

Various methods of CRP determination are available, including nephelometry and turbidimetry.

CRP antibodies reagent with the antigen in the sample and form an antigen-antibody complex. This antigen-antibody complex is measured after agglutination using turbidimetry. PEG is added to reach the end point quickly, increase sensitivity, and minimize the risk of measuring false-negative levels in samples with excess antigen.

The detection sensitivity should be at least 1 mg/l.

Reference range [51]: (The values are consensus values)

mg/dl	mg/l
< 0,5	< 5

CRP in Comparison with Other Acute Phase Reactants

CRP is the most sensitive of the acute phase proteins which can be readily measured in the laboratory. At present there are no clear indications for the determination of other acute phase proteins.

Although almost 30 acute phase proteins are known, only CRP and serum amyloid A (SAA) are suitable as indicators of an acute phase response (APA). Both show a sharp increase shortly after an inflammatory stimulus and, as a result of their short half-life, a rapid drop after disappearance of the stimulus [100].

Rheumatoid Factors (RF)

RF is found in 70-90% of RA. Therefore, a negative result does not rule out a diagnosis of RA, especially if only one determination has been performed. RF often precedes the onset of the illness, sometimes by many years. The risk of RF-positive healthy individuals developing RA is stated to be 5-40 times higher than in RF-negative individuals.

RF is not specific for RA, as it is encounted in many rheumatic and non-rheumatic diseases. In the elderly, the proportion of positive RF findings in the absence of corresponding signs of clnically overt disease increases to as high as 20%. RF is valuable in the differential diagnosis of rheumatological diseases because various diseases which are important from a differential diagnostic point of view, such as psoriasis arthritis, ankylosing spondylitis, gout, reactive arthritides, polymyalgia rheumatica, and arthroses, are not associated with a higher prevalence of RF than in the normal population. Higher titers of RF are more specific for the diagnosis of RA [126].

RF is a heterogenous group of auto-antibodies directed against the antigenic determinants on the Fc portion of IgG molecules. RF is important for the diagnosis of rheumatoid arthritis but can also occur in various non-rheumatic diseases and in clinically healthy individuals over the age of 60. Despite these limitations, detection of RF is one of the diagnostic criteria of the American College of Rheumatology for the detection of rheumatoid arthritis [2]. The auto-antibodies occur in all immunoglobulin classes, but the conventionally used methods are limited to the detection of IgM rheumatoid factor [132].

Methods of Determination

All methods are based on the reaction of RF with antigens, the Fc portion of human or animal IgG. These antigens are employed as aggregates or particle or solid-phase bound in divser assays.

A typical immunological turbidity test is based on the principle of the immunological agglutination test with latex used to amplify the reaction.

Latex-bound, heat-deactivated IgG (antigen) reacts with the antibodies in the sample and form antigen-antibody complexes that are measured after agglutination using turbidimetery.

Reference interval [51]

< 14 IU/ml	< 14 kU/l

Iron/Copper Relation and Ceoruloplasmin

In rheumatological diagnostics, a decrease in serum iron concentration is usually an indication of redistribution of iron in the body to macrophages of the RES (reticuloendothelial system) as part of the chronic inflammation process.

Parallel to this process, the serum copper level almost always increases as a result of increased synthesis of ceruloplasmin, an acute phase protein. The simultaneous determination of Fe and Cu (or ferritin, transferritin saturation, ceruloplasmin) is therefore clinically more useful. While there are many causes of iron deficiency, the inflammatory reaction is usually the only cause of elevated copper levels. An Fe/Cu quotient of < 1, as found in inflammatory-rheumatic diseases, is also observed in other chronic states of infection (ACD). Cp is important for intracellular oxidation of Fe^{2+} to Fe^{3+} which is necessary for release of iron ions from the cells and the binding to transferrin.

References

1. Alford CE, King TTE, Campell PA (1991) Role of transferrin, transferrin receptors and iron in macrophage listericidal activity. J Med 174: 45-9-466
2. Arnett FC, Edworthy SM, Bloch DA et al. (1988) The American Rheumatism Association 1987 revised criteria for the classification of rheumatoid arthritis. Arthritis Rheum, 31: 315-324
3. Arosio P, Levi S, Gabri E et al (1984) Heterogeneity of ferritin II: immunological aspects. In: Albertini A, Arosio P, Chiancone E, Drysdale J (eds) Ferritins and isoferritins as biochemical markers. Elsevier, Amsterdam New York Oxford, pp 33-47
4. Baker EN, Lindley PF (1992) New perspectives on the structure and function of transferrin. J Inorg Biochem 47: 147-160
5. Baynes RD (1994) Iron Deficiency in Iron Metabolism in Health and Disease (eds. Brock JH, Halliday JW, Pippard MJ, Powell LW) W.B. Saunders Co., p. 189
6. Begemann H, Rastetter J (1993) Klinische Hämatologie, 4. Aufl. Thieme, Stuttgart New York
7. Beguin Y (1992) The soluble transferrin receptor: biological aspects and clinical usefulness as quantitative measure of erythropoiesis. Haematologica 77: 1-10
8. Beguin Y et al (1993) Quantitative asessment of erythropoiesis and functional classification of anemia based on measurement of serum transferrin receptor and Erythropoetin. Blood 81: 1067

9. Besarab A, Bolton WK, Browne JK, Egne JC, Nissenson AR, Okamoto DM, Schwab SJ, Goodkin DA (1998) The effect of normal as compared with low hematocrit values in patients with cardiac disease who are receiving hemodialysis and Erythropoetin.N Engl J Med 339: 584 - 590

10. Beutler E (1997) Genetic irony beyond haemochromatosis: clinical effects of HLA-H mutations. Lancet 349: 296-297

11. Bobbio-Pallavicini F, Verde G, Spriano P, Losi R et al (1989) Body iron status in critically ill patients: significance of serum ferritin. Int Care Med 15: 171-178

12. Boelaert JR, Weinberg GA, Weinberg ED (1996) Altered iron metabolism in HIV infection: Mechanisms, possible consequences and proposals for management. Inf Dis Agents 5: 36-46

13. Bothwell TH, Baynes RD, MacFarlane BJ, MacPhail AP (1989)Nutritional iron requirements and food iron absorption. J Intern Med 226: 357-365

14. Brock JH (1994) Iron in infection, immunity, inflammation and neoplasia in Iron Metabolism in Health and Disease; ed Brock JH, Halliday JW, Pippard MJ, Powell LW London, W.B. Saunders, pp 353 -389

15. Brouwer DAJ, Welten HTME et al (1998) Plasma folic acid cutoff value, derived from its relationship with homocyst(e)ine. Clin Chem 44/7: 1545-1550

16. Bunn HF (1991) Anemia associated with chronic disorders. In: Harrison's principles of internal medicine, 12th ed., McGraw-Hill, New York, pp 1529-1531

17. Burns DL, Pomposelli JJ (1999) Toxicity of parenteral iron dextram therapy. Kid Int 55 (Suppl. 69): S 1l9 - S124

18. Cazzola M, Poncho L, Debenedetti F, Ravelli A, Rosti V, Beguin Y, Invernizzi R, Barosi G, Martini A (1996) Defective iron supply for erythropoesis and adequate endogenous Erythropoetin production in anemia associated with systemic onset invenile chronic arthritis. Blood 87; 4824 - 4830

19. Chiancone E, Stefanini F (1984) Heterogeneity of ferritin I structural and functional aspects. In: Albertini A, Arosio P, Chiancone E, Drysdale J (eds) Ferritins and isoferritins as biochemical markers. Elsevier, Amsterdam New York Oxford, pp 23-31

20. Cook JD et al (1993) Serum transferrin receptor. Annu Rev Med 44: 63

21. Cook JD, Skikne BS, Baynes RD (1986) Serum transferrin receptor. Blood 687: 726-731

22. Covell AM, Worwood M (1984) Isoferritins in plasma. In: Albertini A, Arosio P, Chiancone E, Drysdale J (eds) Ferritins and isoferritins as biochemical markers. Elsevier, Amsterdam New York Oxford, pp 49-65

23. Danielson BG, Salmonson T, Derendorf H, Geisser P (1996) Pharmacokinetics of iron(III)-hydroxide sucrose complex after a single intravenous dose in healthy volunteers. Arzneimittelforschung/Drug Res 46 (I) 6

24. De Jong G, von Dijk IP, van Eijk HG (1990) The biology of transferrin. Clin Chim Acta 190: 1-46

25. De Sousa M, Reimao R, Porto G, Grady RW, Hilgartner MW, Giardina P (1992) Iron and lymphocytes: Reciprocal regulatory interactions. Curr Stud Hematol Blood Transf 58: 171 - 177

26. Deinhard AS, List A, Lindgren B, Hunt JV, Chang PN (1986) Cognitive deficits in iron-deficient and iron-deficient anaemic children. J Paediatr 108: 681-689

27. Deutsch E, Gever G, Wenger R (1992) Folsäure-Resorptionstest. In: Laboratoriumsdiagnostik. Wissenschaftliche Buchreihe, Schering, 91

28. Dietzfelbinger H (1993) Korpuskuläre hämolytische Anämien. In: Begemann H, Rastetter J (Hrsg) Klinische Hämatologie, 4. Aufl. Thieme, Stuttgart New York, S 248

29. Dinant JC, de Kock CA, van Wersch JWJ. Diagnostic value of C-reactive protein measurement does not justify replacement of the erythrocyte sedimentation rate in daily general practice. Eur J Clin Invest 1995; 25; 353-9

30. Dorizzi RM, Fortunato A, Marchi G, Scattolo N (2000) Reference interval of ferritin in premenopausal women calculated four laboratories using three different analyzers. Clin Biochem 33: 75-77

31. Drysdale JW (1977) Ferritin phenotypes: structure and metabolism. In: Jacobs A (ed) Iron metabolism. Ciba Foundation Symposium 51 (excerpta medica). Elsevier, Amsterdam, pp 41-57

32. Drapier JC, Hirling H, Wietzerbin H, Kaldy P, Kühn LO (1993) Biosynthesis of nitric oxide activates iron regulatory factor in macrophages. EMBO J 12: 3643-3650

33. Elliot MJ, Maini RN (1994) Repeated therapy with monoclonal antibody to tumor necrosis factor alpha (cA2) in patients with rheumatoid arthritis. Lancet 344: 1125-1127

34. Erslev AJ (1991) Erythropoetin. N Engl J Med 324: 1339-1344

35. Eschbach JW, Haley NR, Adamson JW (1990) The anemia of chronic renal failure: pathophysiology and effects of recombinant Erythropoetin. Contrib Nephrol 78: 24-37

36. Ferguson BJ, Skikne BS, Simpson KM, Baynes RD, Cook JD (1992) Serum transferrin receptor distinguishes the anemia of chronic disease from iron deficiency anemia. J Lab Clin Med 19: 385-390

37. Finch CA, Huebers HA, Cazzila M, Bergamaschi G, Bellotti V (1984) Storage iron. In: Albertini A, Arosio P, Chiancone E, Drysdale J (eds) Ferritins and isoferritins as biochemical markers. Elsevier, Amsterdam New York Oxford, pp 3-21

38. Finlayson NDC (1990) Hereditary (primary) hemochromatosis. BMJ 301: 350-351

39. Flowers CH et al (1989) The clinical measurement of serum transferrin receptor. J Lab Clin Med 114: 368

40. Forman DT, Vye MV (1980) Immunoradiometric serum ferritin concentration compared with stainable bone marrow iron as indices to iron stores. Clin Chem 26: 145-147

41. Franco RS (1987) Ferritin. In: Pesce AJ, Kaplan LA (eds) Methods in clinical chemistry. CV Mosby Company, St. Louis Washington Toronto, pp 1240-1242

42. Garry PJ (1984) Ferritin. In: Hicks JM, Parker KM (eds) Selected analytes in clinical chemistry. American Association for Clincal Chemistry Press, Washington, pp 149-153

43. Goldberg MA, Dunning SP, Bunn HF (1988) Regulation of the Erythropoetin gene: evidence, that the oxygen sensor is a hemo protein. Science 24w: 1412-1415

44. Gottschalk R, Wigand R, Dietrich CF, Oremek G, Liebisch F, Hoelzer D, Kaltwasser JP (2000) Total iron-binding capacity and serum transferrin determination under the influence of several clinical conditions. Clin Chim Acta 293: 127-138

45. Greendyke RM, Sharma K, Gifford FR (1994) Serum levels of erythropoietin and selected cytokines in patients with anemia of chronic disease. Am Clin Path 101: 338-341

46. Grützmacher P, Ehmer B, Messinger D et al (1991) Therapy with recombinant human Erythropoetin (rEPO) in hemodialysis patients with transfusin dependent anemia. Report of a European multicenter trial. Nephrologia 11: 58–65

47. Gunshin H, Mackenzie B, Berger UV, Gunshin Y, Romero MF, Boron WF, Nussberger S, Golan JL, Hediger MA (1997) Cloning and characterization of a mammalian proton-coupled metal-ion transporter. Nature 388: 482–488

48. Haupt H, Baudner S (1990) Chemie und klinische Bedeutung der Human Plasma Proteine. Behring Institut Mitteilungen 86: 1-66

49. Haverkate F, Thompson SG, Pyke SDM, Gallimore JR, Pepys MB (1997) Production of C-reactive protein and risk of coronary events in stable and unstable angina. Lancet 349: 462-466

50. Heidelberger M, Kendall FE (1935) The precipitin reaction between type III pneumococcus polysaccharide and homol-

ogous antibody III. A quantitative study and theory of the reaction mechanism. J Exp Med 61: 563-591

51. Heil W, Koberstein R, Zawta B, Reference Ranges for Adults and Children, Pre-Analytical Considerations. Roche Diagnostics GmbH

52. Heinrich HC (1980) Diagnostischer Wert des Serumferritins für die Beurteilung der Gesamtkörper-Eisenreserven. In: Kaltwasser JP, Werner E (Hrsg) Serumferritin. Springer, Berlin Heidelberg New York, S 58-95

53. Henry DH (1990) Erythropoetin therapy in AIDS. Prog Clin Biol Res 338: 113-120

54. Henry DH, Abels RI (1994) Recombinant human Erythropoetin in the treatment of cancer and chemotherapy-induced anemia: results of double-blind and open label follow-up studies. Semin Oncol 21 [2 Suppl 3]: 21-28

55. Hershko Ch, Konijin AM (1981) Serum ferritin in hematologic disorders. In: Albertini A, Arosio P, Chiancone E, Drysdale J (eds) Ferritins and isoferritins as biochemical markers. Elsevier, Amsterdam New York Oxford, pp 143-158

56. Hörl WH, Cavill I, Cove-Smith R, Eschbach J, Macdougall IC, Salmonson T, Schaefer RM, Sunder-Plassmann G (1995) How to get the best out of r-HuEPO? Nephrol Dial Transplant 10 (Suppl. 2): 92-95

57. Hörl WH, Cavill I, Macdougall IC, Schaefer RM, Sunder-Plassmann G (1996) How to diagnose and correct iron deficiency during rhEPO therapy, a consensus report. Nephrol Dial Transplant 11: 246-250

58. Huber H, Löffler H, Pastner D (1992) Diagnostische Hämatologie – Laboratoriumsdiagnose hämatologischer Erkrankungen, 3. Aufl., Springer, Berlin Heidelberg New York Tokyo

59. Huebers HA, Beguin Y, Pootrakne P, Einspahr D, Finch CA (1990) Intact transferrin receptors in human plasma and their relation to erythropoiesis. Blood 75: 102-107

60. International Committee for Standardisation in Haematology (1985) Proposed international standard of human ferritin for the serum ferritin assay. Br J Haematol 61: 61
61. International Committee for Standardisation in Haematology (1988) Recommendations for measurement of serum iron in blood. Int J Hematol 6: 107-111
62. Jacobs A, Hodgetts J, Hoy TG (1984) Functional aspects of isoferritins. In: Albertini A, Arosio P, Chiancone E, Drysdale J (eds) Ferritins and isoferritins as biochemical markers. Elsevier, Amsterdam New York Oxford, pp 113-127
63. Jacobs A, Worwood M (1975) Ferritin in serum. N Engl J Med 292: 951-956
64. Jazwinska EC et al (1996) Haemochromatosis and HLAH. Nature Genet 14: 249-251
65. Johannsen H, Gross AJ, Jelkmann W (1989) Erythropoetin production in malignancy. In: Jelkmann W, Gross AJ (eds) Erythropoetin. Springer, Berlin Heidelberg New York Tokyo, pp 80-91
66. Johnson AM (1996) Ceruloplasmin. In: Ritchie RF, Navolotskaia O (eds) Serum proteins in clinical medicine. Scarborough: Foundation for Blood Research, 13.01-1-8
67. Jouanolle AM et al (1996) Haemochromatosis and HLA-H. Nature Genet 14: 251-252
68. Kaltwasser IP, Werner E (Hrsg) (1980) Serumferritin: Methodische und klinische Aspekte. Springer, Berlin Heidelberg New York
69. Kaltwasser JP, Werner E (1980) Serumferritin als Kontrollparameter bei der Therapie des Eisenmangels. In: Kaltwasser JP, Werner E (Hrsg) Serumferritin: Methodische und klinische Aspekte. Springer, Berlin Heidelberg New York, S 137-151
70. Kaltwasser JP, Hörl WH, Cavill J, Thomas L (1999) Anaemia, novel concepts in renal and rheumatoid disease, IFCC-Worldlab-Abstracts, Florence

71. Karupiah G, Harris N Inhibition of viral replication by nitric oxide and its reversal by ferrous sulfate and tricarboxylic acid cycle metabolites. J. Exp. Med. 181: 2171-2180

72. Kessler U, Gottschalk R, Stucki G, Kaltwasser JP (1998) Benefit in clinical outcome and disease activity of treatment of anaemia of chronic diseases in rheumatoid arthritis with recombinant human Erythropoetin. J Rheumatol 41: 210

73. Kiechl S, Willeit J, Egger G, Poewe W, Oberhollenzer F (1997) Body iron stores and the risk of carotid atherosclerosis: Prospective results from the Bruneck Study. Circulation 96: 3300-3307

74. Knekt P, Revanen A, Takkunen H, Aromas A, Heliovaara M, Hakulinen T (1994) Body iron stores and the risk of cancer. Int J Cancer 56: 379-382

75. Köhler G, Milstein C (1975) Continuous cultures of fused cells secreting antibody of predefined specificity. Nature 256: 495

76. Kolbe-Busch S, Hermsen D, Reinauer H (2000) Method comparison: Three fully mechanized assays for the quantifiction of the soluble transferrin receptor. Abstract, 52nd AACC, San Francisco

77. Krainer M, Fritz E, Kotzmann H et al (1990) Erythropoetin modulates lipid metabolism. Blut 61: Abstr No 81

78. Kubota K, Tamura J, Kurabayashi H, Shirakura T, Kobayashi I (1993) Evaluation of increased serum ferritin levels in patients with hyperthyroidism. Clin Invest 72 :26-29

79. Leedma PJ, Stein AR, Chin WW, Rogers JT (1996) Thyroid hormone modulates the interaction between iron regulatory proteins and the ferritin mRNA iron responsive element. J Biol Chem 271: 12017-12023

80. Liebelt EI (1998) in Clinical Management of Poisoning and Drug Overdose. WB Saunders 757-766

81. Lindenbaum J (1988) Neuropsychiatric disorders caused by cobalamin deficiency in the absence of anemia or macrocytosis. N Engl J Med 318: 1720-1728

82. Linke R, Küppers R (1989) Nicht-isotopische Immunoassays – Ein Überblick. In: Borsdorf R, Fresenius W, Günzler H et al (Hrsg) Analytiker-Taschenbuch, Bd 8. Springer, Berlin Heidelberg New York Tokyo, S 127-177

83. Linkesch W (1986) Ferritin bei malignen Erkrankungen. Springer, Wien New York

84. Lipschitz DA, Cook JD, Finch CA (1974) A clinical evaluation of serum ferritin as an index of iron stores. N Engl J Med 290: 1213-1218

85. Liuzzo G, Biasucci LM, Gallimore JR et al (1994) The prognostic value of C-reactive protein and serum amyloid A protein in severe unstable angina. N Engl J Med, 331: 417-424

86. Ludwig H, Chott A, Fritz E (1995) Increase of bone-marrow cellurarity during Erythropoetin treatment in myeloma. Stem Cells (Dayton) 13: [Suppl. 2] 77-87

87. Ludwig H, Fritz E, Leitgeb C, Pecherstorfer M et al (1994) Prediction of response to Erythropoetin treatment in chronic anemia of cancer. Blood 84: 1056-1063

88. Ludwig H, Leitgeb C, Pecherstorfer M et al (1994) Recombinant human Erythropoetin for the correction of anemia in various cancers. Br J Haematol 87 [Suppl. 1]: 158 Abstr No 615

89. MacDougall IC, Roberts DE Neu. - A rationale for treatment. Contrib Nephrol 76: 112-121

90. Means RT (1995) Pathogenesis of the anemia of chronic disease: A cytokine mediated anemia. Stem. cells (Dayt) 13: 32-37

91. Means RT, Krantz SB (1992) Progression in understanding the pathogenesis of the anemia of chronic disease. Blood 7: 1639-1647

92. Menacci A, Cenci E, Boelaert JR, Bucci P, Mosci P, Fe'd'Ostiani C, Bistoni F, Romani L (1997) Iron overload

alters T helper cell responses to Candida albicans in mice. J Infect Dis 175: 1467-1476

93. Mercuriali F, Gualtieri G, Sinigaglia L, Inhilleri G, Biffi E, Vinci A, Colotti MT, Barosi G, Lambertenghi Deliliers G (1994) Use of recombinant human Erythropoetin to assist autologous blood donation by anemic rheumatiod arthritis patients undergoing major orthopedic surgery. Transfusion 34: 501-506

94. Mutane J, Piug-Parellada P, Mitjavila MT (1995) Iron metabolism and oxidative stress during acute and chronic phases of experimental inflammation. Effect of iron dextran and desferoxamine. J Lab Clin Med 126: 435-443

95. Nyman M (1959) Serum haptoglobin methodological and clinical studies. Scand J Clin Lab Invest 11 [Suppl. 39]

96. O'Neil-Cutting MA, Crosby WH (1986) The effect of antacids on the absorption of simultaneously ingested iron. JAMA 255: 1468-1470

97. Paruta Sl, Hörl WH (1999) Iron and infection. Kidney International 55 (69), 125-130

98. Peeters HRM et al (1996) Effect of recombinant human Erythropoetin on anaemia and disease activity in patients with rheumatoid arthritis and anaemia of chronic disease: a randomised placebo controlled double blind 52 weeks' clinical trial. Am Rheum Dis 55: 739-744

99. Peeters HRM, Jongen-Lavrencic M, Bakker CH (1999) Recombinant human Erythropoetin improves health-related quality of life in patients with rheumatoid arthritis and anaemia of chronic disease; utility measures correlate strongly with disease activity measures. Rheumatol Int 18: 201-206

100. Pepys MB (1996) The acute phase response and C-reactive protein. In: Weatherall DJ, Kuller LH, Tracy RP, Shaten J, Meilahn EN. Relation of C-reactive protein and coronary heart disease in the MRFIT nested case control study. Am J Epidemiol, 144: 537-547

101. Pincus T et al (1990) Multicenter study of recombinant human Erythropoetin in correction of anemia in rheumatoid arthritis. Am J Med 89: 161-168
102. Pinggera W (1999) Persönliche Mitteilung
103. Ponka P (1999) Cellular iron metabolism. Kidney International, Vol. 55, Suppl. 69, S 2-11
104. Ponka P (1997) Tissue-specific regulation of iron metabolism and heme synthesis: Distinct control mechanisms in erythroid cells. Blood 89: 1-25
105. Ponka P, Beaumont C, Richardson DR (1998) Function and regulation of transferrin and ferritin. Semin Hematol 35: 35-54
106. Punnonen K, Irjala K, Rajamäki A (1994) Iron deficiency anemia is associated with high concentrations of transferrin receptor in serum.Clin Chem 40: 774-776
107. Punnonen K et al (1997) Serum transferrin receptor and its ratio to serum ferritin in the diagnosis of iron deficiency. Blood 89/3: 1052-1057
108. Refsum AB, Schreiner BBI (1984) Regulation of iron balance by absorption and excretion. Scand J Gastroenterol 19: 867-874
109. Richardson DR, Ponka P (1997) The molecular mechanisms of the metabolism and transport of iron in normal and neoplastic cells. Biochem Biophys Acta 1331: 1-40
110. Riedel HD, Fitscher BA, Remus AJ, Stremmel W (1997) Ist das Haemochromatose-Gen identifiziert? Ein neu entdecktes MHC-Klasse-I-Gen mutiert bei Patienten mit hereditärer Haemochromatose. Z Gastroenterol 35: 155-157
111. Ritchey AK (1987) Iron deficiency in children. Update of an old problem. Postgrad Med 82: 59-63
112. Roberts AG et al (1997) Increased frequency of the haemochromatosis Cys 282 Tyr mutation in sporadic prophyria cutanea tarda. Lancet 349: 321-323
113. Robinson SH (1990) Degradation of hemoglobin. In: Williams WJ, Beutler W, Erslev AJ, Lichtman MA (eds) Hematology, 4th edn, McGraw-Hill, New York

114. Rosenberg IH, Alpers DH (1983) Nutrional deficiencies in gastrointestinal disease. In: Sleisenger MH, Fordtran JS (eds) Gastrointestinal disease, 3rd edn, Saunders, New York, pp 1810-1819

115. Roth D, Smith RD, Schulman G et al (1994) Effects of recombinant human Erythropoetin on renal function in chronic renal failure predialysis patients. Am J Kidney Dis 24: 777-784

116. Rowland TW, Kelleher JF (1989) Iron deficiency in athletes. Insights from high school swimmers. Am J Dis Child 143: 197-200

117. Ruggeri G, Jacobello C, Albertini A et al (1984) Studies of human isoferritins in tissues and body fluids. In: Albertini A, Arosio P, Chiancone E, Drysdale J (eds) Ferritins and isoferritins as biochemical markers. Elsevier, Amsterdam New York Oxford, pp 67-78

118. Sandborn WJ, Hanauer SB (1999) Antitumor necrosis factor therapy for inflammatory bowel disease: a review of agents, pharmacology, clinical results and safety. Inflammatory Bowel Diseases 5 (2): 119-133.

119. Sassa S (1990) Synthesis of heme. In: Williams WJ, Beutler E, Erslev AJ, Lichtman MA (eds) Hematology, 4th edn, McGraw Hill, New York, p 332

120. Schultz BM, Freedman ML (1987) Iron deficiency in the elderly. Baillieres Clin Haematol 1: 291-313

121. Schurek HJ (1992) Oxygen shunt diffusion in renal cortex and its physiological link to Erythropoetin production. In: Pagel H, Weiss C, Jelkmann W (eds) Pathophysiology and pharmacology of Erythropoetin. Springer, Berlin Heidelberg New York Tokyo, pp 53-55

122. Scigalla P, Ehmer B, Woll EM et al (1990) Zur individuellen Ansprechbarkeit terminal niereninsuffizienter Patienten auf die Rh-EPO-Therapie. Nieren Hochdruckerkrankungen 19: 178-183

123. Scott JM, Weir DG (1980) Drug induced megaloblastic change. Clin Haematol 9: 587-606

124. Shapiro HM (1995) Practical flow cytometry 3rd ed. New York: Wiley-Liss

125. Stevens RG, Jones DY, Micozzi MS, Taylor PR (1988) Body iron stores and the risk of cancer. N Engl J Med 319: 1047-1052

126. Strant PW (1975) Alkoholwirkung auf das Blut. Schweiz Med Wochenschr 105: 1072

127. Sullivan JL (1996) Perspectives on the iron and heart disease debate. J Clin Epidermial 49: 1345-1352

128. Sunder-Plassmann G, Hörl WH (1996) Eisen und Erythropoetin. Clin Lab 42: 269-277

129. Sunder-Plassmann G, Hörl WH (1999) Erythropoetin and iron. Kidney International 55 (69)

130. Suominen P et al (1997) Evaluation of new immunoenzymometric assay for measuring soluble transferrin receptor to detect iron deficiency in anaemic patients. Clin Chem 43/9: 1641-1646

131. Thomas AJ, Bunker VW, Stansfield MF, Sodha NK, Clayton BE (1989) Iron status of hospitalized and housebound elderly people. Q J Med 70: 175-184

132. Thomas L (Ed.) (1998) Clinical Laboratory Diagnostics, 1st Edition, TH Books Verlagsgesellschaft, Frankfurt

133. Thomas L, Kaltwasser JP, Kuse R, Pinggera W, Scheuermann EH, Wick P (1997) Konsensus Konferenz: Eisensubstitution bei Dialysepatienten unter Erythropoetintherapie. Frankfurt (unveröffentlichte Mitteilung)

134. Thorstensen K, Romslo I (1993) The transferrin receptor: its diagnostic value and its potential as therapeutic target. Scand J Clin Lab Invest 53 [Suppl. 215]: 113-120

135. Thorpe SJ, Walker D, Arosio P, Heath A, Cook JD, Worwood M (1997) International collaborative study to evaluate a recombinant ferritin preparation as an International Standard. Clin Chem 43: 1582-7

136. van Leeuwen MA, van Rijswijk MH, Sluiter WJ et al. (1997) Individual relationship between progression of radiological damage and the acute phase response in early

rheumatoid arthritis. Towards development of a decision support system. J Rheumatol, 24: 20-27

137. Waheed A, Parkkila S, Saarnio J Fleening RE et al. (1999) Association of HFE protein with transferrin receptor in crypt enterocytes of human duodenum. Proc. Nat. Acad. Sci. USA 96: 1579-1584

138. Weiss G (1999) Iron and anemia of chronic disease. Kidney international 55 (69), 12-17

139. Weiss G, Fuchs D, Hausen A, Reibnegger G, Werner ER, Werner Felmayer G, Wachter H (1992) Iron modulates interferon gamma effects in the human myelomonocytic cell line THP-1 Exp Hematol 20: 605-610

140. Weiss G, Houston T, Kastner S, Johrer K, Grunewald K, Brock JH (1997)Regulation of cellular iron metabolism by Erythropoetin: Activation of iron-regulatory protein and up-regulation of transferrin receptor expression in erythroid cells. Blood 89: 680

141. Weiss G, Wachter H, Fuchs D (1995) Linkage of cell-mediated immunity to iron metabolism. Immunol Today 16: 495-500

142. Weiss G, Werner-Felmayer G, Werner ER, Grunewald K, Wachter H, Hentze MW (1994) Iron regulates nitric oxide synthase activity by controlling nuclear transcription. J Exp Med 180: 969

143. Weiss TL, Kavinsky CJ, Goldwasser E (1982) Characterization of a monoclonal antibody to human Erythropoetin. Proc Natl Acad Sci USA 79: 5465-5469

144. Wick M, Pinggera W (1994) (persönliche Mitteilung)

145. Williams WJ, Beutler E, Ersler AJ, Lichtman MA (eds) (1990) Hematology, 4th edn, McGraw-Hill, New York

146. Worwood M (1980) Serum ferritin. In: Cook JD (ed) Methods in hematology. Churchill Livingstone, New York, pp 55-89

147. Yanagawa S, Hirade K, Ohnota H (1984) Isolation of human Erythropoetin with monoclonal antibodies. J Biol Chem 259: 2707-2710

148. Yap GS, Stevenson MM (1994) Inhibition of in vitro erythropoiesis by soluble mediators of Plasmodium chalandi AS malaria: lack of a major role of interleukin l, TNF alpha and gamma-interferon. Infect Immun 62: 357-362

Recommended Reading

Albertini A, Arosio P, Chiancone E, Drysdale J (eds) (1984) Ferritins and isoferritins as biochemicalmarkers. Elsevier, Amsterdam New York Oxford

Begemann H, Rastetter J (1993) Klinische Hämatologie, 4. Aufl. Thieme, Stuttgart New York

Burmester G (1998) Taschenatlas der Immunologie: Grundlagen Labor, Klinik. Thieme, Stuttgart New York

Heil W, Koberstein R, Zawta B (2000) Reference Ranges for Adults and Children, Pre-Analytical Considerations, Roche Diagnostics GmbH, Mannheim

Klein J, Horejsi N(1999) Immunology, 2nd ed., Blackwell Science, Oxford, Malden, Carlton

Thomas L (Ed.) (1998) Clinical Laboratory Diagnostics, 1st ed., TH Books Verlagsgesellschaft, Frankfurt

Beutler E, Lichtman MA, Coller BS, Kipps Th (1995) William's Hematology. 5th ed., McGraw-Hill, New York

Sunder-Plassmann G, Hoerl WH, Guest Editors, (1999), Kidney International, Vol. 55, Suppl. 69

Brostoff J (1997) Taschenatlas der Immunologie: Grundlagen Labor, Klinik. Thieme, Stuttgart New York

Forth W, ed. Iron. (1993) Bioavailability, absorption and utilization. Mannheim, Wissenschaftsverlag

Subject Index

5-desoxyadenosylcobalamin
ACD (anemia of chronic diseases) 75, 109
Aceruloplasminemia 30
Acute phase protein 96, 152, 162
Acute phase reaction 48, 96
Agglutination 150
Alcoholism 42, 74
Anaphylactic reaction 107
Anemias
aplastic 73
chronic 75, 109
corpuscular 97
hemolytic 27, 49, 95
hyperchromic 139
hypochromic 95
infectious 40
macrocytic 89, 97
microcytic 49
normocytic 95, 139
pernicious 93
sideroachrestic 27, 74
sideroplastic 73
therapy 102
tumor anemia 39, 84, 116
uremic 86, 118
in renal failure 118

Anemias of chronic diseases (ACD) 74, 109
Anti-acute phaseprotein 32, 48
Antibody 149
monoclonal 149
polyclonal 149
Antibody excess 151
Antigen excess 151
Antigen-antibody reaction 149
Anti-nuclear antibodies (ANA) 172
Antistreptococcus-desoxyribonuclease titer (ADNse) 172
Anti-streptolysin antibodies (ASL) 172
Anulocytes 66
Apoferritin 11
Apotransferrin 15, 33, 112
Ascorbic acid (Vitamin C) 104
Auto-antibodies 34, 50
cold antibodies 34, 50
warm antibodies 50
Autoimmune diseases 114, 172
Automated cell count 172
Autoregulation, iron metabolism 15, 34

Bantusiderosis 30

Basic isoferritins 13
Basic L-ferritin-subunits 13
Beta-1-trnsferrin-mobility 5
Beta-2- and 1-transferrin 5
Blood count 125
    large (red and white) 125
    small (red) 125, 126
Blood donors 16, 67
Bone marrow 12, 13, 17
Bone marrow infiltration 35
Bone marrow stem cells 18, 82,
    114
Borosolicate glass capillaries 135

C1 units, -carriers 16
Carboxyhemoglobin (COHb) 133
Cardiac muscle 13
Cardiovascular diseases 108
CDT 5
Cerebral sclerosis 28
Cerebral spinal fluid (CFs) 5
Ceruloplasmin 3, 11, 142, 164,
    177
CFU-GEMM (hematopoietic
    stem cells) 82
    chronic diseases (ACD) 34, 83
    chronic renal insufficiency 86,
    118
    tumor anemia 84, 116
Circadian rhythm 7, 147
Classification criteria for RA 172
Classification criteria of anemias
    139
Cobalamin (vitamin B1) 16, 42,
    166

5-deoxyadenosylcobalamin
    166
Cofactors of erythropoiesis 87,
    89, 121, 123
Cold antibodies 50, 95
Combination EPO/iron therapy
    113, 117, 121
Conjugates of glucoronic acid 22
Connective tissue diseases 173
Cook's equation 122
Coombs test 50
Coronary heart disease 27, 108
C-reactive protein (CRP) 113,
    121, 173
    determination 174
Cyanide ions (CN) 134
Cyanmethemoglobin 134
Cytokines 15, 35, 81
Cytotoxic effects 15, 35, 81

DCT 1 (divalent cation trans-
    porter 1) 4, 10, 72
Defects of erythrocyte enzymes
    96
Depot iron 2, 9, 23, 56
Desoxyhemoglobin (HHb) 133
Diabetes mellitus 27
Diagnostic recommendations
    115, 120
Dialysis patients 36, 86, 118
Differential diagnosis 100, 102
    anemis of RA 72
    iron deficiency 65
    macrocytic anemias 89
    normocytic anemias 95
    uremic anemias 86

Dissociation of the vitamin B_{12}-intrinsic factor complex 166
Donath-Landsteiner antibodies 50
Duodenum 4

EDTA blood 127
Endoxidase I (= ceruloplasmin) 3, 11, 142, 164, 177
Enzyme immunoassay 149
Ery survival time, shortened 10, 75
Erythroblasts 17, 19
Erythrocyte indices 137
Erythrocytes 21, 136
  count (RBC) 17, 136
  degradation 10, 21
  maturation 16, 136
  morphology 21, 45
  old 21
Erythrocyte sedimentation rate (ESR) 173
Erythrocytopenia 170
Erythrocytosis 170
Erythropoiesis 16
  co-factors 63, 87
  deficiency 87
  differentation 16
  disturbances 23, 42, 87
  ineffective 27, 86
Erythropoiesis activity 23
Erythropoietin (EPO) 18, 40, 83, 84, 113, 117, 121
  dose 113, 121
  production 40
  therapy 23, 113, 117, 121

tumor markers 84
deficiency 18, 40
EPO/Iron therapy 113, 117, 121
Erythropoietin (EPO) formation 18, 83, 84, 86, 113, 121
  raised 18, 40, 84, 113
  reduced 18, 40, 86, 121
Erythropoietin determination 169
Etanercept79, 110
Excretion of iron ions 29
Extrinsic factor 166

Femtoliter (fl) 137
Ferritin 11, 55, 69, 152
  apoferritin 11
  indicator function 11, 13, 27, 51, 63, 109, 118, 152
  isoferritin (acidic, basic) 11, 13, 152
  non-representative increase 13
  organ-specificity 13
  subunits H, L 11, 152
  synthesis 11
Ferritin, methods of determination 154
  age and gender-dependence 155
  automation 154
  clinical interpretation 56
  ferritin concentration 155
  raised, non-representative 69
  raised, representative 70
  reduced 63
  reference range 155
  representative 56

Ferritin Fe^{3+} 11
Ferritin release 152
Ferrochelatase 46
Ferrous fumarate 104
Ferrous gluconate 104
Ferro sulfate 104
Ferro Zine® 145
Fluorescence immunoassay 149
Folic acid 17, 42, 136, 137, 162
  antagonists 41
  carrier of C1-units 16
  deficiency 40, 90
  deficit 90, 169
  determination 168
  folic acid deficiency, causes
    40, 90, 168
  neurological symptoms 90
  requirement 90, 169
  resorption test 90
  synthesis by intestinal bacteria
    168
  therapy 123
Free Hemoglobin in plasma 133
Functional iron 15, 55
Functional iron deficiency 31, 34

Glucose-6-phosphate-dehydroge-
  nase 50, 96

Haptoglobin 48, 162
  phenotypes 162
Haptoglobin-hemoglobin com-
  plex 162
Hart failure 27
Heidelberger-Kendall curve 151
Hematocrit (Hkt) 135

Hematological diagnostics 125
Hematology analyzer 127
Hemiglobin (Hi) 133
Hemiglobin cyanide method 134
Hemochromatosis 28, 70
  acquired 74
  primary 28, 70
  secondary 38, 73
Hemoglobin (Hb) 17, 21, 42
  degradation 21
  HbA$_0$, A$_2$, Hb Bart's 44
  HbF, HbH, HbS 474
  synthesis 17
Hemoglobin derivatives 133
Hemoglobin measurement, photometric 134
Hemoglobin reference values 134
Hemoglobinopathies 42, 49
Hemoglobin synthesis 17, 44, 46
  2α- and 2δ-chains (HbA2) 17,
    44
  2α- and 2β-chains (HbAO) 17,
    44
  2α- and 2γ-polypeptide chains
    (HbF) 17, 44
  α2-glycoprotein 17, 44
  α-chain thalassemia 17, 44
  α-chains 17, 44
  β-chains 17, 44
  β-lactoglobulin 18, 44
  β-thalassemia 18, 44, 46
  γ-chains 18, 44, 46
Hemoglobinuria 50
Hemolysis 23, 36, 48, 95
  auto-immune 36
  corpuscular 48

extracorpuscular 50
Hemolysis agent 128
Hemopexin 48
Hemosiderin 21
Hemosiderosis 76
HFE gene 28, 71
HFE protein 28, 71
High-dose hook effect 151
HLA-Gen 28
Hodgkin's diease 173
Homocysteine 41
Hyperhomocysteinanemia 41
Hypermenorrhea 16
Hypoferremia 75

IFN-γ, interferon-γ 15, 33, 112
Immune defense 77
Immunoassays 149
    enzyme immunoassays 149
    fluorescence immunoassays
    149
    latex immunoagglutination as-
    says 150
    nephelometric assays 150
    radial immunodiffusion 150
    radioassays 149
    turbidimetric assays 150
Immunochemical methods 149
    false determination
Immunological agglutination test
    149
Immunological-analytical meas-
    uring procedures 149
    direct 150
    indirect 149
Impedance principle 128

Impulse counting per unit of vol-
    ume 129
Impulse image 129
Infections 108, 174
Inflammatory bowel disease 168
Inflammatory processes 116
Infliximab 79, 109
Interferon-γ (INF-γ) 15, 33, 112
Interleukin-1 77
Interleukin-6 15, 33, 77, 112
Intracellular destruction 173
Intrinsic factor 17, 41, 93, 166
Iron 3, 114
    day-to-day fluctuations 147
    deficiency 25
    functional iron 36, 118
    requirement 13
    storage iron 9, 146
    total amount 4, 55, 146
    transport iron 5, 6, 7, 25, 146
Iron administration
    intravenous 104
    oral 103
    side-effects 106
Iron balance 23, 53
    disturbances 23, 53
Iron binding capacity 6, 136,
    142, 148, 157
    latent (LIBC) 6, 136, 142, 148,
    158
Iron binding proteins 4, 5, 8, 10,
    11, 142
    determination 149
Iron deficiency 25, 66
    blood donors 68
    breast feeding 68

causes 68
competitive athletes 69
diet 68
functional 36, 118
growth 68
iatrogenic 68
latent 25, 64, 67
manifest 25, 64, 67
menstruation 64, 68
pregnancy 68
prelatent 25, 64, 67
Iron absorption test 52
Iron deficient anemia 25, 63, 103
Iron determination 144
 iron balance 23, 51, 103
 reference interval 147
 with or without deproteination 144
Iron distribution 1
 disorders 31, 74
 therapy 109
Iron fractions in serum 146
Iron incorporation 7
Iron ions 146
Iron ions due to contamination 146
Iron loss 16
 intestine 16
 perspiration 16
 urine 16
Iron metabolism 3
 auto-regulation 14
 disturbances 23, 74, 84
 iron distribution 13
 iron losses 16
 iron requirement 13

iron resorption 3
iron storage 9
iron transport 5
Iron overload 27, 69
 causes 27, 69
Iron oxidation 144
Iron requirement 13
 blood donors 14
 menstruating women 14
 pregnant women 14
 young people 14
Iron absorption 3, 23, 69
 absorption test 52
 disturbances 23
 raised 23, 69
Iron sacharate 104
Iron storage 10
Iron storage tissues 12
 bone marrow 12
 liver 12
 spleen 12
Iron substitution in dialysis patients 121
Iron substitutions 104, 113, 116, 121
Iron sulfate 104
Iron therapy 102
Iron transport 5
Iron turnover 37
Iron uptake 3, 13, 51
Iron utilization disturbances 35, 84, 118
 therapy
Iron/copper relation 10, 164, 177

Kidney carcinoma 40

Kidney, synthesis organ of EPO 19, 164

Lactoferrin 76
LDH, isoenzymes 95
Lesch-Nyhan syndrome 94
Leukocyte dilution 127
Liver diseases 27, 40
LPS, lipopolysaccharide 15, 33, 112
Lysing agent 129

Macrocytes 39
Macrocytic anemias 89
    medication-induced 89
Macrophages 15, 33, 112
Magnesium hydroxide carbonate 148
Malaria plasmodia 49
Malignancy 108, 117
Mean cell volume of erythrocytes (MCV) 137
Mean cellular hemoglobin concentration of erythrocytes (MCHC) 137
Mean cellular hemologin content of erythrocytes (MCH) 137
Mean platelet volume 138
Met-hemoglobin (Met Hb) 133
Methods of determination 125
Methylmalonic acid 42
Microhematocrit method 135
Monocytes 15, 33, 112
Mucosa cell 14, 93 107
Myelodys plastic syndrome (MDS) 36, 40

Myoglobin 55

N-5-methyltetrahydrofolic acid (MTHFA) 169
Neoplasias, malignant 31
NO (nitrogen oxide) 15, 33, 112
Normoblasts 17
    basophilic 17
    oxyphilic 17
Normocytic anemias 88

Oral Iron preparations 103
Orotic acid metabolism 94
Oxygen radicals 15, 33, 112
Oxygen saturation of hemoglobin 19
Oxygen transport 18
Oxyhemoglobin (O_2Hb) 133

Parenteral administration of iron 104, 113, 116, 121
    dose calculation 105, 122
Parietal cells 7
Particle count 128
Phagocytosis 21
Phagocytosis of old erythrocytes 22
Phenotypes, haptoglobin 156
    Hp 1-1 157
    Hp 2-1 157
    Hp 2-2 157
Phlebotomy 73
Phorphyrin ring of heme 22
Polycythemia vera 40
Porphyrin synthesis disturbances 45

Proerythroblasts 17
Pteridine derivative 168
Pteroylmonoglutaminic acid
    (PGA) 168

Reference range 143
    ceruloplasmin 143, 165
    erythropoietin (EPO) 143, 170
    ferritin 143, 155
    folic acid 143, 169
    hemoglobin 134, 143
    heptoglobin 143, 163
    iron 143, 147
    serum/plasma iron 143, 147
    transferrin 143, 157
    transferrin receptor 143, 162
    transferrin saturation 143, 159
    vitamin B$_{12}$ 143, 167
Renal anemia 36, 86, 118
Resorption of Iron 3, 23, 52
Resorption disturbances
    folate 40, 90, 123
    iron 13, 31, 74, 103
    vitamin B$_{12}$ 40, 92, 123
Reticulocyte count 140
Reticulocytes 18, 139
Reticuloendothelial system
    (RES) 15, 74
Rheumatic diseases 32, 75, 109
Rheumatoid arthritis (RA) 32,
    75, 109, 172
Rheumatoid factors 176
Rheumatological diagnostics 172

Sandwich enzyme immunoassay
    149

Serum amyloid A protein (SAA)
    175
Serum ferritin concentration 152
Serum transferrin receptor, solu-
    ble 8, 60, 159
Serum/plasma iron 144
Sickle cell anemia 44, 62
Sickle cells 44
Side effects of iron therapy 106
Sideroachrestic anemias 27, 44,
    46
Soda lime capillaries 135
Soluble serum transferrin recep-
    tor 8, 60, 159
Stem cell proliferation 18, 39
Stomach secretion 39
Storage iron 9, 23, 51

Tetrahydrofolic acid (THFA) 168
Thalassemia 73
    major 73
    minor 73
Therapeutic approaches in ane-
    mias 103
    ACD (anemia of chronic dis-
    ease) 109
    erythropoietin deficiency 118
    folic acid deficiency 123
    iron deficiency 103
    oral administration of iron 103
    parenteral administration of
    iron 104
    RA (rheumatoid arthritis) 109
    renal failure 118
    tumor-induced anemias 116
    vitamin B$_{12}$ deficiency 123

Therapy of anemias 103
Tissue hypoxia 19
TNF-α (tumor necrosis factor a) 15, 33, 112
Transcobalamin 166
Transferrin and TEBK 158
Transferrin concentration 157
Transferrin Fe^{3+} complex 5, 156
Transferrin receptor
Transferrin receptor determination 159
Transferrin anti-acute phase protein 32, 48
Transferrin, apotransferrin 156
Transferrin, methods of determination 156
Transport capacity, iron 6
Trivalent iron in ferritin 146

Trivalent iron in transferrin 146
Tumor anemias 84, 116
Tumor necrosis factor a (TNF-a) 15, 33, 112

Venous thrombosis 165
Vitamin B_6-deficiency 36
Vitamin B_{12} 166
   deficiency 92
   determination 166
   requirement 92
   resorption 94

Warm antibodies 95
WHO criteria of anemias 103

Zinc-protoporphyrin 35, 46
Zollinger-Ellison-Syndrome 94

SpringerMedizin

Wolf-Rüdiger Külpmann,
Hans-Krister Stummvoll,
Paul Lehmann

Elektrolyte

Klinik und Labor

Zweite, erweiterte Auflage
1997. VIII, 164 Seiten. 40 Abbildungen.
Broschiert DM 39,–, öS 275,–
ISBN 3-211-82975-X

In diesem Buch werden die medizinische Bedeutung der Elektrolyte und ihre Bestimmung behandelt. Auf diese Weise wird dem Kliniker ermöglicht, Einblick auch in die Analytik der Elektrolyte zu gewinnen. Die im Labor Tätigen erhalten einen Überblick über Physiologie und Pathologie des Elektrolythaushalts.

Das Buch beschreibt im ersten Teil komprimiert den aktuellen Stand der Diagnose und Therapie von Störungen im Elektrolythaushalt und bietet dem Arzt sowohl eine rasche Orientierungshilfe am Krankenbett, als auch eine vertiefende Einsicht in pathophysiologische Zusammenhänge. Ein besonderer Abschnitt befaßt sich mit den Elektrolyten im Urin.

In den anschließenden Kapiteln werden Präanalytik und Analytik der Elektrolyte unter besonderer Berücksichtigung der Bestimmung mittels ionenselektiver Elektroden sowie „enzymatischer" Methoden und trägergebundener Reagenzien („Trockenchemie") einschließlich der Qualitätssicherung besprochen.

 SpringerWienNewYork

A-1201 Wien, Sachsenplatz 4–6, P.O.Box 89, Fax +43.1.330 24 26, e-mail: books@springer.at, **www.springer.at**
D-69126 Heidelberg, Haberstraße 7, Fax +49.6221.345-229, e-mail: orders@springer.de
USA, Secaucus, NJ 07096-2485, P.O. Box 2485, Fax +1.201.348-4505, e-mail: orders@springer-ny.com
EBS, Japan, Tokyo 113, 3–13, Hongo 3-chome, Bunkyo-ku, Fax +81.3.38 18 08 64, e-mail: orders@svt-ebs.co.jp

SpringerMedicine

Helmut Schenkel-Brunner

Human Blood Groups

Chemical and Biochemical Basis of Antigen Specificity

Second, completely revised edition
2000. XV, 637 pages. 173 figures.
Hardcover DM 198,–, öS 1386,–
(recommended retail price)
ISBN 3-211-83471-0

This monograph covers the entire field of blood group serology, with its main emphasis on the chemical and biochemical basis of blood group specificity. Full consideration is given to molecular biology investigations, in particular to studies on the structure of blood group genes and the molecular biological basis of alleles and rare blood group variants, whereby relevant literature up to the year 2000 is covered.

The text is supplemented by numerous illustrations and tables, and detailed reference lists. The five years since the publication of the first edition have brought further advances in blood group research. Thanks to modern molecular biology, scientists have not only been able to identify the bearer molecules of many more blood groups, they have clarified the molecular basis of a number of further blood group specifities as well.

This book offers a concise survey for use by blood bankers and researchers in biochemistry, blood group serology, immunohematology, forensic medicine, population genetics, and anthropology.

SpringerWienNewYork

A-1201 Wien, Sachsenplatz 4–6, P.O.Box 89, Fax +43.1.330 24 26, e-mail: books@springer.at, **www.springer.at**
D-69126 Heidelberg, Haberstraße 7, Fax +49.6221.345-229, e-mail: orders@springer.de
USA, Secaucus, NJ 07096-2485, P.O. Box 2485, Fax +1.201.348-4505, e-mail: orders@springer-ny.com
EBS, Japan, Tokyo 113, 3–13, Hongo 3-chome, Bunkyo-ku, Fax +81.3.38 18 08 64, e-mail: orders@svt-ebs.co.jp